title of the book indicates, I have attempted to present those
methods which are used in the analysis of epidemiological studies. For
s, this was a hazardous undertaking. One reason is that it is still a
field. The book naturally reflects my own appraisal of what is relevant
lopments hitherto. I am aware that others might make different
d that I myself may in some cases have misunderstood the biostatisti-
will be very grateful for your views on these issues—both large and

of the hazards I faced was that it was my intention to write a book
read without any prior knowledge of statistics, even while some of
described here can be considered relatively advanced, (for example
ulating exact confidence intervals). A consequence of this is that the
irly narrow focus. It only takes up those aspects of the underlying
d statistical theories which are necessary for epidemiological
e it goes into those specific methods in some depth.
f my intention to write a work which does not demand prior
re is no doubt that a basic understanding of statistics and epidemiol-
ading of the book much easier.
an be seen as the third part of a trilogy, the two previous parts of
ntroduction to epidemiology (Ahlbom & Norell: *Introduction to
iology*, Epidemiology Resources, Inc., 1990) and a book about the
iological studies (Norell: *A Short Course in Epidemiology*, Raven

and foremost like to thank Staffan Norell for our longstanding
for the many constructive and stimulating discussions which were
nce in the shaping of this book. I would also like to extend a
Lars Alfredsson for his many valuable opinions about the various
uscript and for an appendix with exercises which significantly
e of the book. Arne Bjurman, Niklas Hammar, Göran Pershagen,
Gunnar Steineck, Åke Svensson and Magnus Wickman have all
le views and comments on the various stages of the manuscript,
e owed many thanks. Lastly, I would like to thank Jennifer
admirable courage, threw herself and her word processor into
athematical formula.
would like to thank Judith Black for translating the Swedish
k into English. A challenging task for a literature scientist.

BIOSTATISTICS
for
EPIDEMIOLOGISTS

Anders Ahlbom

Karolinska Institute
Stockholm, Sweden

Appendix with exercises and solutions by Lars Alfredsson

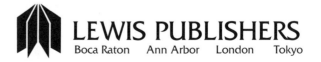

LEWIS PUBLISHERS

Boca Raton   Ann Arbor   London   Tokyo

To G E S P

Library of Congress Cataloging-in-Publication Data

Catalog record is available from the Library of Congress

ISBN 0-87371-912-3

PRINTED IN THE UNITED STATES OF AMERICA
1 2 3 4 5 6 7 8 9 0

Printed on acid-free paper

THE AUTHOR

Anders Ahlbom is currently Professor and Head of the Department of Epidemiology at the Institute of Environmental Medicine, Karolinska Institute. He has previously published the *Introduction to Modern Epidemiology* now available in six languages. Professor Ahlbom's experience is from teaching epidemiology and biostatistics in Europe and the United States.

CONTENTS

Chapter 1

INTRODUCTION

"Vital statistics and their analysis are essential features of public health work, to define its problems, to determine, as far as possible, cause and effect, and to measure the success or failure of the steps taken to deal with such problems. They are fundamental to the study of epidemiology."

Hill AB: Principles of Medical Statistics. The Lancet Limited, 1967 (First edition 1937).

Epidemiology is the study of the occurrence of disease. The occurrence of disease is studied in relation to factors relating to the individual, his environment and his lifestyle with the aim of establishing the causes of disease. The interpretation of an epidemiological study must always take the validity and the precision of the study into consideration. How one assesses the validity of an epidemiological study is discussed in books on the methodology of epidemiology (see the reference section at the end of this book), while the issue of precision is addressed in books on biostatistics. Biostatistics also includes methods which enable one to take systematic errors, such as the influence of other factors, into account when one is analyzing data, as well as methods for studying the effects of the interaction of risk factors.

The field of biostatistics covers the statistical methods used in biological and medical research. This is a very wide field and strictly speaking does not exclude any area of statistical methodology. In this book we limit ourselves to methods used in epidemiology. Thus the methods are discussed in an epidemiological context and the examples used are from the field of epidemiology. This is not to say that these methods do not have applications in other

1

fields, such as in survival analysis, evaluation of clinical trials or studies of health care use.

The aims of this book are threefold. The first is to provide a collection of methods which can be used to analyze data in most epidemiologic studies. In other words, one should be able to use the book as a statistics handbook or maybe "cookbook" for epidemiology. The second aim is to give an understanding of the theoretical background to the methods described here. With this we hope to demonstrate what the methods can actually achieve and the assumptions upon which they are based. For this reason, the book contains a number of derivations of formulae or, where this would carry too far, some principles as to how derivations could be carried out. The third aim of the book is to discuss some general principles which apply to the analysis of epidemiological data and how the precision of an epidemiologic study can best be described. One example of this is the discussion of the role of significance testing.

The book consists of three parts. The first is preparatory and features a summary of those aspects of the theory of probability which are of importance for the statistical theory which is then taken up. This part of the book also contains a discussion about statistical inference in general and a discussion about statistical inference in epidemiological research in particular. The second part of the book describes the most important methods used for analyzing epidemiological data. It begins with an analysis of descriptive data and goes on to discuss the analysis of effect measures, i.e. measures used to compare exposed and unexposed. This is done firstly without taking any background factors into consideration, then when doing so—in other words crude and stratified analysis. The final part of this section takes up more specific areas. Multivariate models, dose-response analysis, analysis of the interaction between causes of disease, meta-analysis and computer programs are all discussed here.

NOTE: In the examples featured in the text and in the exercises in Appendix 2, the results are generally given with 3-digit accuracy. When relevant, intermediate results are given with four digits accuracy but the calculations have been carried out on the computer which always used maximum accuracy.

Chapter 2

PROBABILITY THEORY

"When they saw a random relationship between what goes into a system and what comes out, they assumed that they would have to build randomness into any realistic theory. The modern study of chaos began with the creeping realization in the 1960s that quite simple mathematical equations could model systems every bit as violent as a waterfall....In weather, for example, this translates into what is only half-jokingly known as the Butterfly Effect — the notion that a butterfly stirring the air today in Peking can transform storm systems next month in New York."

Gleick J: Chaos. Making a New Science. Viking Penguin, Inc., 1987.

One of the main objectives of the statistical analysis of a collected material is to determine the importance of the study's random errors. What can we conclude about the "true" value from an obtained study result? Our conclusions are based on what is known about the probability of different results given different assumptions about the "true" values. Probability theory forms the basis for these calculations.

In this chapter we will go through some of the basic concepts used in probability theory which are of particular importance for the applications discussed in this book. For a more comprehensive presentation of these concepts, we recommend a textbook on this subject, such as one of those referred to in the reading list at the end of the book.

2.1 SOME BASIC PRINCIPLES

The *probability* of an event, E, for example that a randomly chosen person has diabetes, is written $P(E)$ and is a number between 0 and 1, where $P(E) = 0$ when E is impossible and 1 when E is sure to occur. If E_1 and E_2 are two events which cannot happen at the same time, then the probability of at least one of them occurring is $P(E_1) + P(E_2)$.

The *complementary* event to E is denoted as E^* and is the alternative to E. In other words, it is what happens when E does not happen. If E is defined as a randomly chosen person having diabetes, then E^* means that the person in question does not have diabetes. Since either E or E^* always happens:

$$P(E) + P(E^*) = 1$$

Two events, E_1 and E_2, occurring simultaneously is described as E_1E_2 and the probability of this is thus $P(E_1E_2)$. When

$$P(E_1E_2) = P(E_1)P(E_2)$$

E_1 and E_2 are said to be *independent*.

EXAMPLE:

Let the probability of a person randomly chosen from the population having diabetes be 0.02. The probability of two persons both having diabetes will then be 0.0004 provided the condition that they are chosen randomly and independently of each other.

The occurrence of at least one of two events, E_1 and E_2, is denoted as E_1UE_2 and the probability of this is therefore $P(E_1UE_2)$. This probability can be calculated as:

$$P(E_1UE_2) = P(E_1) + P(E_2) - P(E_1E_2)$$

where the last term compensates for the "double counting" which takes place when both E_1 and E_2 occur.

EXAMPLE:

The probability of at least one of the two persons in the previous example having diabetes is $0.02 + 0.02 - 0.0004 = 0.0396$.

On those occasions when E_1 and E_2 are *disjunctive*, i.e., when they cannot occur simultaneously and consequently $P(E_1E_2) = 0$, the formula is simplified to

$$P(E_1UE_2) = P(E_1) + P(E_2)$$

EXAMPLE:

Define E_1 as (exact) one of two persons having diabetes and E_2 as both having the disease. E_1 and E_2 are disjunctive and $P(E_1UE_2)$ is calculated according to the above formula: $P(E_1) = 2 \times 0.02 \times 0.98 = 0.0392$, that is, twice the probability that the first person has diabetes but not the second. One multiplies by two because it could also be the second person who had diabetes while the first did not. $P(E_2) = 0.02 \times 0.02 = 0.0004$ as was shown earlier. The probability of at least one of the two persons having diabetes is therefore $0.0004 + 0.0392 = 0.0396$. Since the alternative to at least one of the two persons having diabetes is that neither of them has the disease in question, the probability can also be calculated as:

$$1 - P(\text{no one has diabetes}) = 1 - 0.98 \times 0.98 = 0.0396$$

Conditional probability means the probability of an event occurring provided that another event has occurred, i.e., the probability of an event under certain conditions. The probability of E_1, on the condition that E_2 has occurred, is written as $P(E_1 | E_2)$ and is calculated as:

$$P(E_1|E_2) = P(E_1E_2)/P(E_2)$$

The denominator can be understood as the normation required since the possible outcomes have been limited by the condition.

EXAMPLE:

The probability of both of the individuals in the example having diabetes, if at least one of them has the disease, is 0.0004/0.0396 = 0.0101.

In the case of independent occurrences, the conditional probability can be written as:

$$P(E_1|E_2) + P(E_1)P(E_2)/P(E_2)$$

which simplifies to $P(E_1|E_2) = P(E_1)$: That is, for independent events the conditional probability is the same as the nominal probability.

2.2 STOCHASTIC VARIABLES

2.2.1 What is a Stochastic Variable?

A variable whose value is determined by the outcome of a random event is called a *stochastic variable*.

EXAMPLE:

If an individual is randomly chosen from a population and a variable X is defined as having the value 1 if the individual has diabetes and 0 otherwise, then X is a stochastic variable.

NOTE: In this chapter, capitals are used to denote stochastic variables and lower case letters for the values which the variable assumes. To comply with accepted epidemiological notations, this distinction is made in a slightly different way in following chapters where we deal explicitly with epidemiological applications.

A stochastic variable which can only assume a finite number of values within a limited interval is said to be *discrete*. Variable X in the above example can only assume the values 0 and 1 and is consequently an example of a discrete stochastic variable.

A discrete stochastic variable is specified by its *probability function*. This is a function which, for each value of the variable, gives the probability of that value being assumed. The probability function can either be given as a table of possible values and corresponding probabilities or as a mathematical formula which gives the corresponding probability for each value of the variable.

EXAMPLE:

Two individuals are randomly and independently chosen from a population where 0.02 have diabetes. The stochastic variable X is defined as the number of persons with diabetes. The probability function, $p(x)$, will be:

x	$p(x)$
0	0.9604
1	0.0392
2	0.0004
Total	1.0000

The probabilities are derived from previous calculations. Note that the sum of all probabilities is 1.

A *continuous variable* can, within a limited interval, take an infinite number of values and the probability for each individual outcome is 0. Therefore, in the case of continuous variables one talks not of probability function but rather of *frequency function*.

NOTE: This illustrates an apparent paradox, namely that the probability of an event being 0 does not mean that the event is impossible.

The probability of a continuous stochastic variable assuming a value within a certain interval is calculated as the integral of the frequency function over the interval.

EXAMPLE:

If a continuous stochastic variable is defined in such a way that it can only assume values between 0 and 1 and that the probability of it assuming a value within an interval (between 0 and 1) is directly proportional to the length of the interval, then the variable is uniformly distributed with the frequency function $f(x)$:

x	$f(x)$
$0 < x \leq 1$	1
otherwise	0

Note that

$$\int_0^1 f(x)\ dx = \int_0^1 1\ dx = 1$$

For discrete as well as for continuous stochastic variables, the distribution function, $F(x)$, is defined as:

$$F(x) = P(X \leq x)$$

For a discrete stochastic variable, $F(x)$ is calculated as the sum of the probability function's values for all values that are less than or equal to x. In the same way, $F(x)$ for a continuous stochastic variable is calculated as the integral of the frequency function over all values less than or equal to x.

EXAMPLE:

The distribution function of the discrete variable whose probability function was described above can be calculated as follows:

x	$p(x)$	$F(x)$
0	0.9604	0.9604
1	0.0392	0.9996
2	0.0004	1.0000

EXAMPLE:

The distribution function for the continuous variable in the example will be:

x	$f(x)$	$F(x)$
$x \leq 0$	0	0
$0 < x \leq 1$	1	x
$1 < x$	0	1

When a stochastic variable is specified with the help of the probability-, frequency, or distribution function, it is said that one is giving the variable's distribution or distribution form.

2.2.2 Mean and Variance

The mean and variance for stochastic variables are defined analogously with how they are defined in descriptive statistics:

The *mean* of the stochastic variable X, $E(X)$, is defined as:

$$E(X) = \sum_x p(x)x \quad \text{or} \quad E(X) = \int_{-\infty}^{\infty} f(x)x\,dx$$

depending on whether the variable is discrete or continuous.

EXAMPLE:

For the discrete variable in the above example one obtains:

$$E(X) = 0.9604 \times 0 + 0.0392 \times 1 + 0.0004 \times 2 = 0.0400$$

EXAMPLE:

Correspondingly, the mean in the example with the continuous variable will be:

$$E(X) = \int_0^1 x\,dx = 0.500$$

Variance, var(X), is defined as the mean of the squared differences between the value of the variable and mean of the variable, i.e., for a discrete variable as:

$$var(X) = \sum_x p(x)[x - E(X)]^2$$

and for a continuous variable as:

$$var(X) = \int_{-\infty}^{\infty} f(x)[x - E(X)]^2 \, dx$$

The variance can also be written as:

$$var(X) = E(X^2) - [E(X)]^2$$

which in connection with certain calculations and derivations is an advantage.

EXAMPLE:

The variance for the discrete variable in the above example will be:

$$var(X) = 0.9604 \times (0 - 0.0400)^2 + 0.0392 \times (1 - 0.0400)^2 +$$
$$+ 0.0004 \times (2 - 0.0400)^2 = 0.0392$$

EXAMPLE:

The example with the continuous variable gives:

$$var(X) = \int_0^1 (x - 0.500)^2 \, dx = 0.0833$$

2.2.3 Transformations

Later in the book we will form new stochastic variables from one or several previously defined variables by so-called *transformations*. In the case of certain transformations one can calculate the mean and variance of the newly-formed variables from the corresponding parameters for the original variables.

One very commonly used transformation is the so-called *linear combination*. If a stochastic variable X is defined as:

$$X = a_0 + a_1 X_1 + ... + a_k X_k$$

where X_1, ..., X_k are stochastic variables and $a_0, a_1, ..., a_k$ are constants, then X is said to be a linear combination of the stochastic variables X_1, ..., X_k. It is easy to show that:

$$E(X) = a_0 + a_1 E(X_1) + ... + a_k E(X_k)$$

Provided that X_1, ..., X_k are independent, it is also easy to show that:

$$var(X) = a_1^2 \, var(X_1) + ... + a_k^2 \, var(X_k)$$

NOTE: Independence between stochastic variables is defined analogously with the independence of events in a random trial. However, for a more exact definition we refer the reader to a textbook on probability theory.

EXAMPLE:

Let us look again at the two randomly chosen individuals from the population with 0.02 diabetics. Define X_1 as 1 if the first individual has diabetes and as 0 otherwise, and define X_2 as 1 if the second individual has diabetes and as 0 otherwise. Now define a new variable as:

$$X = X_1 + X_2$$

i.e., as the number of diabetics; this is a linear combination where both the a-constants in front of the original variables are 1.

Both the mean and the variance for this variable were calculated earlier in this chapter from the probability function. We shall now see that the same result is obtained if the above formulae are used. The mean for the two variables is obtained directly from the definition of the mean:

$$E(X_1) = E(X_2) = 0.0200 \times 1 + 0.9800 \times 0 = 0.0200$$

The mean of the new variable will be, according to the formula for the mean of linear combinations:

$$E(X) = 1 \times 0.0200 + 1 \times 0.0200 = 0.0400$$

This agrees with what was obtained when the calculations were based on the probability function.

X_1 and X_2 are independent stochastic variables, or at least they are such if the population is so large that the proportion of diabetics is not affected by one diabetic being removed from the population. $Var(X)$ can therefore be calculated by using the formula for linear combinations given previously if $var(X_1)$ and $var(X_2)$ are known. These are calculated directly from the definition as:

$$var(X_1) = var(X_2) = 0.02 \times (1 - 0.02)^2 + 0.98 \times (0 - 0.02)^2 =$$

$$0.02 \times 0.98 = 0.0196$$

$var(X)$ is therefore:

$$0.0196 + 0.0196 = 0.0392$$

which also agrees with the previous calculations.

EXAMPLE:

For another example of this type of transformation, let $Y = X/2$, i.e., the proportion of diabetics among the two chosen individuals. Y is formed here from a single variable, X, and the a-constant in front of this is $1/2$. The mean and the variance are thus respectively:

$$E(Y) = 1/2 \times E(X) = 1/2 \times 0.0400 = 0.0200$$

and

$$var(Y) = (1/2)^2 \times var(X) = (1/2)^2 \times 0.0392 = 0.0098$$

We will also sometimes come across transformations which are not linear. The most important of these is the *logarithm transformation*. In a logarithm transformation each value of a variable is substituted by its logarithm. By logarithm here we mean the natural logarithm; the one which has the mathematical constant $e \approx 2.718$ as base. This logarithm is denoted as ln. Thus, in a logarithm transformation the variable X is transformed into a variable Y so that $Y = \ln X$; the logarithm is taken for each value that X can assume to give the corresponding value of the variable Y. (Many calculators have a logarithm function with which this can easily be performed.) If $x = 2$ then $\ln x = \ln 2 = 0.6931$. One can reobtain the original value as follows by taking the so-called antilogarithm or by exponentiating:

$$e^{0.6931} = 2.718^{0.6931} = 2$$

$e^{0.6931}$ is often written as $exp(0.6931)$ for typographical reasons. (Calculators which have a logarithm function usually also have an exponential function which can be used here.)

EXAMPLE:

Let a variable, X, have the values 1, 2 and 3 each with the probability $1/3$. If this variable is transformed to the variable Y using $Y = \ln X$, variable Y will take the values $\ln1 = 0$, $\ln2 = 0.6931$ and $\ln3 = 1.099$ each with the probability 1/3:

x	y	p
1	0	1/3
2	0.6931	1/3
3	1.099	1/3

In the case of non-linear transformations there are no simple, general ways of transforming the original variance so that it is valid for the new variable. It is however possible to obtain good approximations.

One method is based on writing the transformed variable as a polynom with terms in rising potency according to a mathematical method which is called the Taylor expansion and on the assumption that terms of higher order can be left out (Armitage, 1971; page 97). If $Y = f(X)$ where X is a stochastic variable and f a function which transforms each X-value to a Y-value, then:

$$var(Y) \approx \left[\frac{dY}{dX}\right]^2 var(X)$$

where dY/dX is calculated for $E(X)$ or for an estimate thereof.

We will often use this in connection with the logarithm transformation. If $Y = \ln X$ then:

$$\frac{dY}{dx} = \frac{1}{X}$$

The variance for Y is consequently:

$$var(Y) \approx \left[\frac{1}{E(X)}\right]^2 var(X) = \frac{var(X)}{[E(X)]^2}$$

In other words, the variance for a variable obtained through the logarithm transformation is obtained by dividing the original variance by the square of the mean.

EXAMPLE:

If we assume that the mean and the variance of variable X are both 10, then for the variable $Y = \ln X$:

$$var(Y) \approx \frac{var(X)}{[E(X)]^2} = \frac{10}{10^2} = \frac{1}{10}$$

2.3 SOME DISTRIBUTIONS

The previous section of this chapter looked at the distributions for a number of stochastic variables. It is clear that there is no limit to the number of this type of distribution. However, some have proven to be more useful than others, and these have been studied closely by statisticians and mathematicians; they have often also got names. For the applications described in this book there are four types of distribution which are particularly important; we will now look at each of these.

2.3.1 The Normal Distribution

The *normal distribution* is a continuous stochastic variable. It is defined by the frequency function:

$$f(x) = \frac{1}{\sqrt{2\pi var(X)}} \exp\left[-\frac{(x - E(X))^2}{2var(X)}\right]$$

The normal distribution is symmetrical around its mean and unlimited both downwards and upwards. The frequency function is specified by the two *parameters* $E(X)$ and $var(X)$, i.e., by the mean and the variance.

If a normally distributed variable is subjected to a linear transformation, the new variable is also normally distributed but the mean and the variance are influenced by the transformation in the way described in the previous section. If X is a normally distributed variable and Z is defined as:

$$Z = \frac{X - E(X)}{\sqrt{var(X)}}$$

then Z is consequently also normally distributed. The mean and the variance of Z are then $E(Z) = 0$ and $var(Z) = 1$. This normal distribution is called the *standardized normal distribution*. The standardized normal distribution will be shown to be very important, and for the sake of simplicity Z will be reserved for variables which follow this distribution.

To indicate that a stochastic variable is normally distributed one usually writes:

$$X \sim N[E(X), \ var(X)]$$

where what is inside the brackets are the parameters which specify how the specific normal distribution looks. The fact that Z follows the standardized normal distribution is consequently written as:

$$Z \sim N(0, \ 1)$$

Even if the normal distribution has attractive mathematical characteristics it cannot be integrated without using special tricks, and calculating the probability of an outcome within a specific interval is complicated. However, there are comprehensive tables for the standardized normal distribution and there are also programs for calculators and personal computer's which can calculate the desired probabilities. If the specific normal distribution is not standardized it must be standardized before the tables or programs can be used. (See Figure 2.1).

EXAMPLE:

A table of the standardized normal distribution shows, for example, that $P(Z > 1.645) = 0.050$. In the same way, $P(X > 5.290) = 0.050$ if $X \sim N(2, 4)$. To see this the following transformation is performed:

$$z = (5.290 - 2)/\sqrt{4} = 1.645$$

If one wants to establish the value of x when $P(X > x) = 0.025$, one uses a table or calculator to arrive at $P(Z > 1.960) = 0.025$.

It thus follows that:

$$X = 2 + 1.960 \times \sqrt{4} = 5.920$$

The normal distribution is probably the most frequently used of all distributions. This is because of a combination of two conditions. First, the normal distribution, in spite of the inaccessible form of the frequency function, has attractive mathematical properties which has meant that a very great number of statistical methods have been developed for applying to normally distributed variables or variables derived from the normal distribution. Second, many variables in application situations are approximately normally distributed. This is not primarily because biological and other variables per se tend to be normally distributed but rather because of the so-called *Central Limit Theorem*. This is a theorem which, in simple terms, says "If observations from sufficiently large materials with independent observations are added together, the sum is approximately normally distributed, regardless of the distributions from which the observations originate." This means, for example, that the mean of a random sample or an incidence rate can often be treated as an observation of an approximately normally distributed variable.

In the case of the applications we deal with in this book, the variables we are interested in are usually the number of cases of disease or some function of this. The probability functions for these variables are, however, infeasible to calculate with large materials, and in such cases the normal distribution can often be used instead as an approximation. This approximation is sometimes considerably improved if the original variable is first transformed so that it becomes less asymmetric. Logarithm transformation is frequently used for this purpose, but other transformations are also used.

2.3.2 The Binomial Distribution

Let X be a stochastic variable which assumes the value 1 with probability p and the value 0 with probability $1 - p$. Such a variable is said to be *dichotomous*. Dichotomous variables are used to describe random events which either "succeed" or "fail." Dichotomous variables are used, for example, to describe disease versus no disease. Earlier in this chapter we had an example of a dichotomous variable which was defined as 1 if an individual had diabetes and 0 otherwise.

The mean and variance for a dichotomous variable is calculated directly from the definitions:

$$E(X) = p \times 1 + (1 - p) \times 0 = p$$

and

$$var(X) = p(1 - p)^2 + (1 - p)(0 - p)^2 = p(1 - p)$$

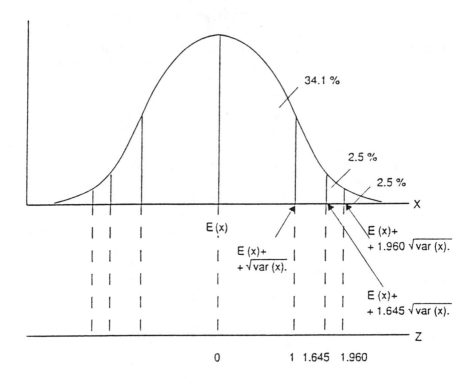

Figure 2.1   The frequency function for a normally distributed variable *X* with mean value *E*(*X*) and variance *var*(*X*). Some probabilities are indicated. The figure illustrates the relationship between an original and a standardized, normally distributed variable. The standardized variable has been achieved by the transformation:

$$Z = \frac{X - E(X)}{\sqrt{var(X)}}$$

If X_1 ,,, X_n are *n* independent stochastic variables which are all distributed as above, then:

$$X = X_1 + \ldots + X_n$$

is *binomially distributed*. The distribution varies depending on the probability, p, and the number of terms in the sum, n. Thus the binomial distribution is: specified by the two parameters n and p. From here on, a variable X which is binomially distributed with parameters n and p will be written $X \sim bin(n, p)$.

The binomial distribution is used to describe the number of "successful trials" in a series of trials carried out independently and under identical conditions, and a binomially distributed variable can assume the values 0, 1, ..., n. The binomial distribution is used to describe, for example, how many individuals in a population have fallen ill with a disease.

EXAMPLE:

In the earlier example, where two individuals were randomly chosen from a population, the number with diabetes can be seen as a binomially distributed variable with the parameters $n = 2$ and $p = 0.02$.

When the outcomes of n independent dichotomous variables, all with the parameter p, are observed, the probability that the first x observations should equal 1 and the other remaining $(n - x)$ observations equal 0 is $p^x(1 - p)^{(n - x)}$. This is also the probability for every other outcome with x 1:s and $(n - x)$ 0:s. The probability for x 1:s is therefore $p^x(1 - p)^{(n - x)}$ multiplied by the number of possible outcomes with x 1:s. This number is (pronounced "n over x"):

$$\binom{n}{x} = \frac{n!}{x!(n - x)!} = \frac{n(n - 1)(n - 2)...1}{x(x - 1)...1(n - x)(n - x - 1)...1}$$

For a full explanation of this we would refer the reader to a text book in probability theory, but $n! = n(n - 1) ... 1$ is the number of ways in which the n different observations can be ordered, while $x!$ and $(n - x)!$ is the number of ways in which the 1:s and the 0:s respectively, can be ordered. The probability function of the binomial distribution is therefore:

$$p(x) = \binom{n}{x} p^x (1 - p)^{(n - x)}$$

With the help of a little algebra it can be shown that $p(x)$ fulfills the condition:

$$\sum_{x=10}^{n} p(x) = 1$$

(See Figure 2.2.)

EXAMPLE:

If X is the number of diabetics in the earlier example, where two individuals are chosen randomly and independently, then $X \sim bin(2, 0.02)$. Although we have already calculated the various values of the probability function earlier, we repeat this here to illustrate how the probability function of the binomial distribution is used:

$$p(0) = \binom{2}{0}0.02^0(1 - 0.02)^{(2 - 0)} = 1 \times 1 \times 0.98^2 = 0.9604$$

$$p(1) = \binom{2}{1}0.02^1(1 - 0.02)^{(2 - 1)} = 2 \times 0.02 \times 0.98 = 0.0392$$

$$p(2) = \binom{2}{2}0.02^2(1 - 0.02)^{(2 - 2)} = 1 \times 0.02^2 \times 1 = 0.0004$$

Since the binomial distribution is obtained as the sum of a number of dichotomous variables, the formulae for the mean and variance of the binomial distribution are obtained by the rules applying to linear combinations:

$$E(X) = np \text{ and } var(X) = np(1 - p)$$

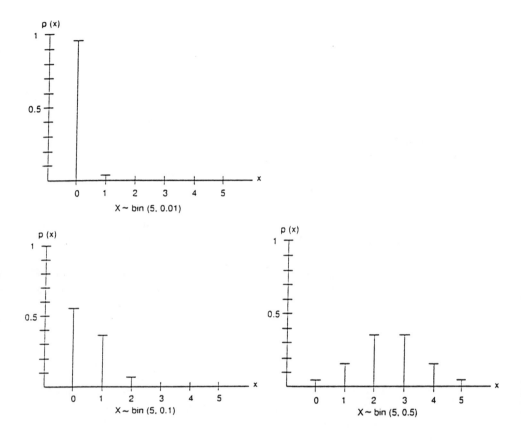

Figure 2.2   The probability function for three binomially distributed variables with $n = 5$ and $p = 0.01$, 0.1 and 0.5 respectively. The figure illustrates how the asymmetry is altered when p changes.

EXAMPLE:

In the above example,

$$E(X) = 2 \times 0.002 = 0.04$$

and

$$var(X) = 2 \times 0.02 \times (1 - 0.02) = 0.0392$$

The formula for the probability function of the binomial distribution is difficult to use in the case of large materials, i.e., with large n. On the other hand, the normal distribution can be used for approximation and the approximation improves as the size of the material, that is n, increases. As was demonstrated earlier, the normal distribution is a symmetrical distribution, while the binomial distribution is only symmetrical when $p = 0.5$. The approximation thus becomes better the nearer p is to 0.5. In epidemiological applications, where p corresponds to a cumulative incidence or a prevalence, p is often very small, and considerable material is then needed for the approximation of the normal distribution. In such situations, however, one can use an alternative method, the Poisson distribution which will be described later.

The normal approximation is obtained by calculating the mean and the variance of the binomial distribution, which are then used as parameters in the normal distribution.

EXAMPLE:

To illustrate how the normal distribution can be used to approximate a binomial distribution, define the stochastic variable $X \sim bin(20, 0.1)$ and consider $P(X \le 3)$. This probability can be calculated exactly from the probability function as:

$$p(X \le 3) = p(0) + p(1) + p(2) + p(3) =$$

$$= 0.1216 + 0.2702 + 0.2852 + 0.1901 = 0.867$$

To obtain a normal distribution approximation one first calculates:

$$E(X) = 20 \times 0.1000 = 2.000 \text{ and}$$

$$var(X) = 20 \times 0.1000 \times 0.9000 = 1.800$$

which are used as parameters in the normal distribution. Thus, approximately, $X \sim N(2.000, 1.800)$ and

$$P(X \leq 3) \approx P\left(Z \leq \frac{3 - 2.000}{\sqrt{1.800}}\right) = 0.772$$

where Z again is for the standardized normal distribution and where the probability is determined from a table or with the aid of a program for a computer.

The binomial distribution is discrete and can only assume natural numbers, while the normal distribution is continuous and can assume all real numbers. The approximation can therefore be improved by the value 3 in the binomial distribution being represented by the whole interval (2.5-3.5) in the normal distribution. We then get the following approximation:

$$P(X \leq 3) \approx P\left(Z \leq \frac{3.5 - 2.000}{\sqrt{1.800}}\right) = 0.868$$

which should be compared with the exact probability which was calculated as 0.867.

2.3.3 The Poisson Distribution

Consider a situation where an event can occur at any moment during an interval of time and where the probability of an event occurring during a sub interval is directly proportional to the length of the sub interval, and further is independent of how many events have occurred earlier and the length of time that has elapsed since the last event occurred. In this situation the number of events occurring during the interval of time follows the *Poisson distribution*.

The Poisson distribution is a discrete distribution where all the numbers from 0 and up can be assumed. The probability function of the Poisson distribution is:

$$p(x) = \frac{e^{-\mu} \mu^x}{x!} \quad \text{for} \quad x = 0, 1, \ldots$$

This expression can be derived from the probability function for the binomial distribution. One lets the n of the binomial distribution go toward infinity and its p toward zero, but in such a way that np is constant; np then becomes the μ parameter of the Poisson distribution.

Since, with the Taylor expansion e^μ can be written as:

$$e^\mu = \frac{\mu^0}{0!} + \frac{\mu^1}{1!} + \frac{\mu^2}{2!} + \ldots = \sum_{x=0}^{\infty} \frac{\mu^x}{x!}$$

it follows that:

$$\sum_{x=0}^{\infty} p(x) = 1$$

As is demonstrated by the probability function, the Poisson distribution is specified by the single parameter μ and we will use the notation:

$$X \sim \text{Poisson}(\mu)$$

for Poisson distributed variables. The mean for the Poisson distribution is calculated as follows:

$$E(X) = \sum_{x=0}^{\infty} \frac{e^{-\mu} \mu^x}{x!} x = \mu$$

The variance is calculated with the aid of the above and the alternative variance formula as:

$$var(X) = E(X^2) - [E(X)]^2 = \sum_{0}^{\infty} \frac{e^{-\mu} \mu^x}{x!} x^2 - \mu^2 = \mu$$

That is, the mean and the variance of the Poisson distribution are both equal to the distribution's parameter μ.

The Poisson distribution is limited downward by 0 but unlimited upward and is consequently asymmetric. When the parameter μ increases, the asymmetry diminishes.

In epidemiology the Poisson distribution is used in connection with person years rather than persons. The number of person years is regarded as a constant and as an interval of time during which a new case of disease can occur at any time. To use the Poisson distribution in such situations, one lets the incidence rate multiplied by the number of person years, i.e., the expected number of cases of disease, correspond to the parameter of the Poisson distribution. Conversely, this means that parameter μ (the expected number of cases) divided by the number of person years corresponds to the incidence rate. (See Figure 2.3.)

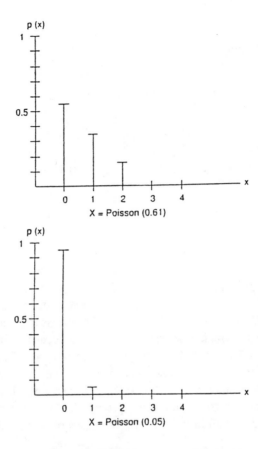

Figure 2.3   The probability function for two Poisson distributed variables with μ = 0.61 and 0.05. The first Poisson distribution is derived from an example described by Fisz (1963). In 10 Polish army units observed over a period of 20 years, the number of deaths resulting from being kicked by a horse were noted. The total number of observations was 200. The average number of deaths per year and army unit was 0.61. If the number of deaths is Poisson distributed, one obtains the distribution described in the figure. Fisz compared this theoretical distribution with the observed one and found that they agreed very closely. As a matter of fact, the theoretical and the observed distributions would not be distinguishable if drawn in the same figure of this type. The second Poisson distribution, with μ = 0.05, can be compared with the first of the three binomial distributions in this figure. The comparison illustrates how a binomial distribution can be approximated with a Poisson distribution.

EXAMPLE:

Let $X \sim$ Poisson(3). Probabilities can then be calculated from the above probability function. Thus, for example:

$$P(X \leq 2) = p(0) + p(1) + p(2) =$$

$$= \frac{e^{-3}3^0}{0!} + \frac{e^{-3}3^1}{1!} + \frac{e^{-3}3^2}{2!} =$$

$$= 0.0498 + 0.1494 + 0.2440 = 0.423$$

EXAMPLE:

As an example with relevance to epidemiology, let us consider a population of 1,000 individuals who are all observed for one year—that is, the study base includes 1,000 person years. Let us assume that the "theoretical" or "true" incidence rate for acute myocardial infarction in the population is 5 per 1,000 person years. The number of cases of myocardial infarction during one year, X, can then be taken as an observation of a Poisson distributed variable with the parameter $\mu = 1,000 \times 0.005 = 5$. This can be used to calculate the probability of various outcomes. For example, the probability of ten or more cases of myocardial infarction is:

$$P(X \geq 10) = 0.0181 + 0.0082 + 0.0034 +$$

$$+ 0.0013 + ... = 0.032$$

With large x values, it becomes difficult to use the Poisson distribution's probability function. However, in such cases the distribution can be approximated by using the normal distribution. To obtain a good approximation, μ should not be too small.

EXAMPLE:

If, in the above example, the normal distribution is used as an approximation, where $\mu = 5$, then:

$$P(X \geq 10) \approx P\left(Z \geq \frac{10 - 5}{\sqrt{5}}\right) = 0.013$$

The approximation can be improved by taking into account the fact that the number of cases must be a natural number. This is achieved by letting the whole interval from 9.5 to 10.5 represent the outcome 10. If one does this, one obtains instead:

$$P(X \geq 10) \approx P\left(Z \geq \frac{9.5 - 5}{\sqrt{5}}\right) = 0.022$$

There are also other ways of obtaining approximations for Poisson distributions. A very good one is described in Rothman and Boice (1982).

With binomial distributions where n is very large and p very small, the normal distribution does not offer a good approximation for the binomial distribution. In this situation, the Poisson distribution can be used instead. When p is small then $np \approx np(1 - p)$ and one of the characteristics of the Poisson distribution, namely that the mean and the variance are the same, is at least approximately satisfied. A binomially distributed variable can assume all natural numbers from 0 to n, while the Poisson distribution can assume all natural numbers from 0 and upwards. Where n is large and p is small, this difference is negligible.

EXAMPLE:

Consider a cohort of 10,000 persons where the cumulative incidence during a follow-up period is 0.0002. If X is the number of cases of disease, it is natural to use the binomial distribution and $X \sim bin(10,000, 0.0002)$. The probability of getting 3 or more cases is then:

$$P(X \geq 3) = 1 - P(X \leq 2) = 1 - p(0) - p(1) - p(2) =$$

$$= 1 - 0.1353 - 0.2707 - 0.2707 = 0.323$$

If one uses a Poisson distribution approximation instead one obtains:

$$X \sim \text{Poisson}(2), \text{ because } E(X) = 10{,}000 \times 0.0002 = 2$$

Then:

$$P(X \geq 3) = 1 - 0.1353 - 0.2707 - 0.2707 = 0.323$$

The normal distribution approximation gives instead 0.362.

2.3.4 The Hypergeometric Distribution

The following example is often used to describe the hypergeometrical distribution. In an urn containing two different types of marble, a certain number of marbles are randomly selected and not returned before the next is picked out. If a stochastic variable is defined as the number of selected marbles of one type, then this is hypergeometrically distributed. If one denotes the stochastic variable as X, then the probability function is:

$$p(x) = \frac{\binom{N_1}{x}\binom{N_0}{n - x}}{\binom{N_1 + N_0}{n}} \quad \max(0, n - N_0) \leq x \leq \min(n, N_1)$$

where N_1 and N_0 are the number of marbles of the two types and n the number of selected marbles. For the epidemiologic applications we have in mind, a different kind of introduction to the hypergeometrical distribution is more natural. Let two independent stochastic variables be distributed as follows:

$$X \sim bin(n_1, p) \text{ and } Y \sim bin(n_2, p)$$

Both the binomial distributions have thus the same p. Consider:

$$X | (n = X + Y)$$

that is, the value of the first of the binomially distributed variables given a certain value on their total. The conditional probabilities are derived from the probability function for the binomial distribution and the formula for conditional probabilities (see Section 2.1), which gives the same results as above.

Observations of hypergeometrical distributions can effectively be presented in the following kind of fourfold table:

	One type of marbles	The other type of marbles	Total
Selected marbles	x	$n - x$	n
Left in the urn	$N_1 - x$	$N_0 - (n - x)$	$N - n$
Total number of marbles	N_1	N_0	N

In epidemiology, the hypergeometrical distribution is used to compare an observed number of events in two populations, usually the number of diseased or the number of exposed people.

EXAMPLE:

Assume that in a population of 5 individuals there are no cases of disease and that in another population of 4 individuals there are 2 cases of disease. Let the number of diseased persons in the two populations be represented by two independent binomial distributions. If one assumes that the risk of becoming diseased is the same in the two populations, the number of diseased persons in the first population, given the total number of cases of disease is hypergeometrically distributed. The data can be presented in a fourfold table as follows:

Disease	Population 1	Population 2	Total
Yes	0	2	2
No	5	2	7
Total	5	4	9

The probability of the observed outcome is:

$$p(0) = \frac{\binom{5}{0}\binom{4}{2}}{\binom{9}{2}} = \frac{1 \times \dfrac{4\times3\times2\times1}{2\times1\times2\times1}}{\dfrac{9\times8...\times2\times1}{7\times6...\times2\times1\times2\times1}} = \frac{1}{6}$$

The hypergeometrical distribution too can be approximated by the normal distribution. The mean and the variance are obtained from the formulae:

$$E(X) = N_1 n/N$$

and

$$var(X) = N_1 N_0 n(N - n)/[N^2(N - 1)]$$

and are used as parameters in the normal distribution.

EXAMPLE:

Consider the table below, set out as in previous examples:

Disease	Population 1	Population 2	Total
Yes	1	5	6
No	4	5	9
Total	5	10	15

Let X be the number of persons with the disease in population 1. Exact probability calculations are performed from the probability function for the hypergeometrical distribution. For example:

$$P(X \leq 1) = p(0) + p(1) = \frac{\binom{5}{0}\binom{10}{6}}{\binom{15}{6}} + \frac{\binom{5}{1}\binom{10}{5}}{\binom{15}{6}} =$$

$$= 0.0420 + 0.2517 = 0.294$$

To obtain a normal distribution approximation one first calculates:

$$E(X) = \frac{5 \times 6}{15} = 2.000$$

and

$$var(X) = \frac{5 \times 10 \times 6 \times 9}{15^2 \times (15 - 1)} = 0.8571$$

In the same way as before one now obtains:

$$P(X <+ 1) \approx P\left(Z \leq \frac{1 - 2.000}{\sqrt{0.8571}}\right) = 0.140$$

As with the previous distributions, the approximation can be improved by taking into account the fact that the normal distribution is continuous. One then gets instead:

$$P(X \leq 1) \approx P\left(Z \leq \frac{1.500 - 2.000}{\sqrt{0.8571}}\right) = 0.295$$

which can be compared with the exact probability of 0.294.

NOTE: The exact probability in the example is used in a statistical procedure called *Fisher's exact test* and the approximate probability agrees in principle with the one obtained by so-called *chi-square tests* for fourfold tables.

The two binomial distributions which were used to define the hypergeometrical distribution had different n but the same p. If the p-values were also different one would instead obtain a *non-central hypergeometrical distribution* (Breslow and Day 1980), the probability function of which is:

$$p(x) = \frac{\binom{N_1}{x}\binom{N_0}{n-x} OR^x}{\sum_i \binom{N_1}{i}\binom{N_0}{n-i} OR^i}$$

where

$$OR = \frac{p_1/(1-p_1)}{p_0/(1-p_0)}$$

and is called the odds ratio. This distribution is used in so-called exact analysis of fourfold tables and is used primarily in exact analyses of data from case-control studies.

Chapter 3

STATISTICAL INFERENCE

"Inductive inferences start with observations of the machine and arrive at general conclusions."

Pirsig RM: Zen and the Art of Motorcycle Maintenance. Vintage, 1991.

Statistical inference means that conclusions about a value in a population are drawn from a random sample or that conclusions about a theoretical value, a *parameter*, in a probability model are drawn from an observed outcome. To be able to talk about statistical inference, the inference must be obtained according to certain principles of which the reliability can be ascertained.

NOTE: *Scientific inference* consists of drawing conclusions about general circumstances from a study result. This makes use of the result of the statistical inference, but also takes into account the systematic errors of the study and the available theoretical information which can be used to assess the potential for drawing general conclusions from the studied population.

In descriptive epidemiologic studies one looks at the occurrence of disease in a particular population during a certain period or at a point in time. One can in such cases maintain that the incidence rate observed describes an entire population and that there is consequently no random uncertainty. No statistical inference would be needed here. However, if the number of cases is under a certain size it is clear that one cannot expect exactly the same incidence rate during an ensuing period of time, and that there is a certain "random" variation between different time periods. This view does not essentially contradict a deterministic view of how diseases develop. One should rather regard the random variations in the occurrence of disease as an expression of variations in the occurrence of risk factors for the disease which for the moment are not known or even suspected. If we may, for a moment, refer to another topical field of research, namely chaos research, this shows that small changes in conditions or initial values can give completely unpredictable results even in simple deterministic models (Gleick 1987).

The magnitude of the "random" variation in the occurrence of disease can be evaluated with the aid of statistical inference. One precondition for this is an *underlying* or *theoretical measure* of the occurrence of disease which is *estimated* from an observed measure of disease occurrence.

The same applies with analytical or aetiological epidemiologic studies where the relationship between a possible risk factor and the occurrence of disease are under study. Conclusions about an underlying theoretical relationship are drawn from observed data.

The chief justification for carrying out empirical studies is the belief that these underlying theoretical relationships or processes do actually exist. If epidemiologic studies were used exclusively to describe the population which is actually under study, their value would be severely restricted.

NOTE: Henceforth, the theoretical, underlying parameters will be given with capital letters. The incidence rate, for example, will be written as I and the ratio between two incidences as RR (as in relative risk or rate ratio). Estimates of these parameters will be written with $\wedge$ on top (pronounced hat). Observed values of these estimates are written in the same way as the estimates, except for when there is a risk of confusing these two; when this is the case the difference is marked in a special way.

Chapter 4

THE P-VALUE, THE P-VALUE FUNCTION AND THE CONFIDENCE INTERVAL

"...reminds me of the number P that I invented a couple of years ago. P is, for each individual, the number of minutes per month that that person spends thinking about the number P. For me, the value of P seems to average out at about 2. I certainly wouldn't want it to go much above that! I find it crosses my mind most often when I'm shaving."

Hofstadter DR: Metamagical themas: Questing for the Essence of Mind and Pattern. Bantam Books 1985.

In medical research, not least in epidemiology, *significance testing* has come to play a very major role; it is often the test result alone which is used to decide whether or not a result is to be ascribed to a random variation. One of the theses in this book is that this is an unsuitable principle, not only because it is fairly uninformative but also because it can easily lead to erroneous conclusions. The present chapter nevertheless begins by discussing the *P-value*, which is the basis not only for significance testing but also for its suggested alternative, the *confidence interval*.

4.1 THE P-VALUE

4.1.1 What is the P-value?

Let us assume that a stochastic variable has a distribution which is determined by a particular parameter and that we have a hypothesis about the

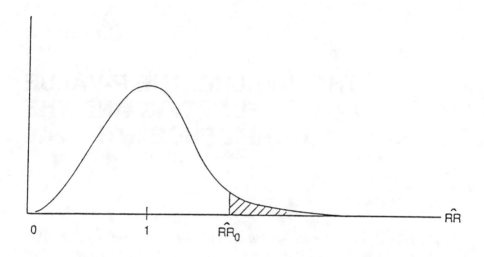

Figure 4.1   The frequency function for the observed relative risk, assuming that the theoretical relative risk, $RR = 1$. The P-value is the probability of getting a value which is at least as large as the observed, that is:

$$P = P(\hat{RR} \geq \hat{RR}_0 | RR = 1)$$

value of that parameter. Sometimes this is called the null hypothesis to distinguish it from other hypotheses. An example of a hypothesis from the field of epidemiology is estimation of the theoretical relative risk. This is done with the help of the observed relative risk, which is a stochastic variable whose distribution depends on the theoretical relative risk. A common hypothesis is that the theoretical relative risk equals 1, in other words, that there is no association between exposure and disease. For each observation on the stochastic variable, the *P-value* is the probability of obtaining an outcome which is at least as extreme as the one which is actually observed, provided that the hypothesis is correct.

EXAMPLE:

Let us assume a hypothesis postulating that a theoretical relative risk equals 1 and the relative risk observed in a study equals 2. The P-value is then the probability of observing a relative risk that is greater or equal to 2 in a new study of the same design. (See Figure 4.1.)

NOTE: The P-value described above is sometimes called *one-sided*. The term *two-sided P-value* refers to the probability of obtaining an outcome that is at least as extreme as the observed outcome, regardless of whether the deviation is upwards or downwards. Since we do not need to use two-sided P-values we shall always refer to one-sided P-values here. See, for example, Armitage (1971) for further discussion.

4.1.2 Some Examples of How to Calculate P-values

EXAMPLE:

Let us assume a hypothesis according to which the prevalence of diabetes in a population is 0.02 and that two individuals are chosen at random from that population. The number of diabetics, A, among these two persons can then be regarded as a binomially distributed variable where $n = 2$ and, according to the hypothesis, $p = 0.02$. If both of the chosen individuals prove to be diabetics, $A = 2$ and the P-value is consequently $P = P(A = 2) = 0.02^2 = 0.0004$. Note that there is no outcome more extreme than the observed one. If, instead, $A = 1$, then $A = 2$ is a more extreme outcome and

$$P = P(A \geq 1) = P(A = 1) + P(A = 2) =$$

$$= \binom{2}{1} 0.02^1 0.98^1 + 0.0004 = 0.0396$$

EXAMPLE:

Let us now assume instead that 100 individuals are selected from a population, with the hypothesis that the prevalence of hypertension is 0.1.

The number of affected persons, A, is once again binomially distributed, this time with $n = 100$ and, according to the hypothesis, $p = 0.1$. In this situation, the P-values can be calculated by normal distribution approximation. Thus, let

$$A \sim N(100 \times 0.1,\ 100 \times 0.1 \times 0.9)$$

If, for example, $A = 15$:

$$P = P\left(Z \geq \frac{14.5 - 10}{\sqrt{9}}\right) = 0.067$$

EXAMPLE:

Let us now consider a situation where the theoretical incidence rates in two populations are the same, with A_1, R_1 and I_1 being the number of cases, number of person years and incidence rate in one population and let A_0, R_0, and I_0 have the corresponding meaning in the other. In each of the populations, the number of cases is regarded as a Poisson-distributed stochastic variable with a parameter which is the product of the number of person years and the theoretical incidence rate. The observed incidence rate is calculated as:

$$\hat{I}_i = \frac{A_i}{R_i},\ \text{for } i = 0,\ 1$$

and is regarded as a stochastic variable. When there is a sufficiently large expected number of cases, $I_i \times R_i$, a normal distribution approximation can be used to determine the probabilities. To calculate a P-value for the hypothesis that the two incidence rates agree, the following stochastic variable is formed:

$$\frac{A_1}{R_1} - \frac{A_0}{R_0} \sim N\left(I_1 - I_0,\ \frac{A_1}{R_1^2} + \frac{A_0}{R_o^2}\right)$$

where $I_1 - I_0 = 0$ according to the hypothesis. In the above formula, the variance has been estimated by making separate estimates for the two individual populations. However, the hypothesis specifies a subsidiary condition for the variance by stipulating that the two incidence rates must agree. This could be used by instead estimating the variance by combining the two materials.

Let us now assume that in the first population of 1,000 persons 25 cases are observed over one year, while in the other population there are 10 cases per 500 persons in one year. In such a case:

$$P = P\left(Z \geq \frac{\dfrac{25}{1000} - \dfrac{10}{500}}{\sqrt{\dfrac{25}{1000^2} + \dfrac{10}{500^2}}}\right) = 0.268$$

EXAMPLE:

Let us now consider a situation in which the cumulative incidence, that is the probability of becoming ill, is compared for two populations. The number of cases in the two populations can be seen as two binomially distributed variables and the hypothesis is that the parameter p is the same for both distributions. This situation can be analyzed by comparing the two binomial distributions. If the material permits a normal distribution approximation, the analysis is analogous with that of the previous example, the only difference being that the basis of the approximation is the binomial rather than the Poisson distribution, as in the previous example. (An analysis which does not use the normal distribution approximation is more complicated in this kind of situation.)

There is, however, an alternative to this approach, namely so-called *conditional analysis*. This is based on the hypergeometric distribution and on the assumption that the number of cases in the two populations can be assumed to follow two independent binomial distributions, which under this hypothesis have the same parameter, *p*. When the hypothesis is true, the number of cases in one population, given the total number of cases, is hypergeometrically distributed. (See Section 2.3.4.) This means, in the example outlined above, that with a certain total number of cases of illness from two populations, the number of these originating in one of the populations is hypergeometrically distributed, given the hypothesis that the probability of becoming ill is the same for both populations.

The advantage of using the conditional probability distribution is that the probabilities of falling ill do not have to be estimated; as long as these are not of interest in themselves but only in relation to each other, they constitute what is usually called "nuisance" parameters.

Let us once again use the example from Chapter 2, where one person in a population of five becomes ill and five in a population of ten. The number of persons falling ill in each of these populations can be seen as binomially distributed, with $n = 5$ in the first case and $n = 10$ in the second. The hypothesis is that the parameter p is the same in the two populations. A P-value can be based on these two binomial distributions, possibly by using a normal distribution approximation.

Conditional analysis instead uses the fact that a total of six cases of illness have arisen in the two populations and that the number of these originating from, say, the first population, is hypergeometrically distributed if the hypothesis about the identical probabilities of falling ill is correct. The P-value can then be calculated exactly or using the normal distribution approximation. With normal distribution approximation one obtains:

$$P = \left(Z \leq \frac{1.5 - \dfrac{5 \times 6}{15}}{\sqrt{\dfrac{5 \times 10 \times 6 \times 9}{15 \times 15 \times (15 - 1)}}} \right) = 0.295$$

We will return to the conditional approach later, where it will be shown that this often facilitates considerably less complicated analyses because "nuisance" parameters can be eliminated.

4.1.3 Interpretation of the P-value

There are two possible ways of interpreting a low P-value. The first is that an unlikely outcome, i.e., an outcome with low probability, has resulted. The other is that the P-value is based on incorrect assumptions, i.e., that the parameter values of the hypothesis were not correct. A low P-value therefore indicates that the hypothesis is not consistent with the data and should be rejected.

In the field of medicine, a well-established practice has been developed for interpreting P-values, according to which the hypothesis is rejected when P is below 0.05. The result is then said to be (statistically) significant or the difference is (statistically) established. Sometimes an asterisk is used to indicate that P is in the interval 0.001-0.05; two asterisks mark the interval 0.001-0.01 and three asterisks the interval < 0.001.

This kind of use of the significance concept leads to study results falling into two distinct groups: significant and non-significant. This is appropriate in situations where decisions are to be based on study results, and indeed the hypothesis testing theory has primarily been developed for use in decision-making. An example of the application of the significance concept in this way is quality control in production processes, where certain tolerances are specified and determine when the process shall be interrupted for adjustment.

However, the situation is different in epidemiologic and other types of scientific study. To start with, the five-percent limit, like every other limit set in advance, is entirely arbitrary, and it is impossible to explain why $P = 0.051$ should lead to a radically different conclusion from $P = 0.049$. Secondly, a sharp division between significant and non-significant results is not desirable in a scientific context. Decisions about a particular course of action are made after taking all the available empirical and theoretical knowledge into account, never simply from the results of one single study. The conclusion "significant" or "non-significant" is not suitable in this kind of procedure; the pooling of all the available knowledge needs to be based on more informative, quantitative variables.

Neither can the actual P-value be used in this process. The first reason for this is that the P-value depends not only on the strength of the association but also on the size of the study. A large study gives a smaller P-value than a smaller study, all else being equal. The P-value does not enable us to distinguish between the effect of the strength of the association and the effect of the size of the study.

A more important reason for why the actual P-value is unsuitable is that the information contained in the P-value refers only to the null hypothesis. The P-value gives the extent to which the null hypothesis is consistent with the observed outcome, but not how consistent alternative hypotheses are with the outcome. The P-value can therefore only be used to reject the null hypothesis, not to choose an alternative. In other words, if the hypothesis concerns the relative risk, a low P-value is interpreted as indicating that the relative risk is not equal to 1.00. However, the P-value says nothing about whether 1.10 is consistent with the outcome, or whether one has to go up to 10.0 to find RR values consistent with the observed outcome.

The P-value is often wrongly understood as the probability that the hypothesis is correct, yet it cannot possibly be interpreted in this way, since the P-value is calculated under the assumption that the hypothesis is correct. Much of the popularity of the P-value seems to be founded on this misunderstanding.

It is thus clear that significance testing, in the form described here, should not be used for analyzing epidemiologic data. This does not, of course, mean that one should disregard random variations, but rather that one should use other methods than the P-value and significance testing. A number of works addressing this question are included among the references (for example, *The Lancet* (editorial) 1987; Langman 1986; Rothman 1978; Walker 1986).

4.2 THE P-VALUE FUNCTION

4.2.1 What is the P-value Function?

The P-value shows how consistent the observed outcome is with the hypothesis. In the contexts we discuss here, this generally means that the P-value carries information about how consistent the observed data are with the hypothesis that there is no association between exposure and disease, i.e., that $RR = 1.00$. The P-value, however, says nothing about how consistent the observed material is with other hypotheses, for example, that $RR = 1.10$ or that $RR = 10.0$. Under some conditions, (for example when the study is large), the outcome can thus be inconsistent with the hypothesis that $RR = 1.00$ but at the same time wholly consistent with the hypothesis that $RR = 1.10$. This is a quite different situation from one where the result is not only inconsistent with the hypothesis that $RR = 1.00$ but also with the hypothesis that $RR = 10.0$. The P-value can thus not be used to decide which parameter values are compatible with the outcome of the study.

It seems reasonable to extend the P-value to a *P-value function*, which gives the probability of a more extreme outcome not only for the parameter value of the null hypothesis, but also for other parameter values (Miettinen 1985; Poole 1987). This means, when considering the relative risk RR, that:

$$P = \begin{cases} P(\hat{RR} \geq \hat{RR}_0 | RR) & \text{when } \hat{RR}_0 > RR \\ P(\hat{RR} \leq \hat{RR}_0 | RR) & \text{otherwise} \end{cases}$$

shall be calculated assuming that $RR = 1.00$, as before, but also with a number of other assumptions about RR. These calculations show how consistent the observed outcome is with a series of RR values, and from this one can decide which RR values are likely in the light of the study results. (See Figure 4.2.)

4.2.2 Two Examples

EXAMPLE:

To illustrate this principle, let A, the number of cases of illness in a *study base* (population studied over a certain time), follow a Poisson distribution with unknown parameter μ ($\mu = I \times R$, where I is the incidence rate and R is the number of person years). If $A = 2$ observed cases of illness occur, the P-value can be calculated for any value of μ:

$$P = P(A \geq 2|\mu) = \sum_{x=2}^{\infty} e^{-\mu}\,\mu^x/x! \quad \text{for } \mu < 2$$

and

$$P = P(A \leq 2|\mu) = \sum_{x=0}^{2} e^{-\mu}\,\mu^x/x! \quad \text{for } \mu > 2$$

The following table can be calculated on the basis of the above:

P	0.005	0.018	0.025	0.037	...	0.062	0.030	0.025	0.014
μ	0.100	0.200	0.242	0.300	...	6.00	7.00	7.22	8.00

The table gives a number of values for the relevant P-value function. The table shows, for example, that if $\mu = 0.100$ then $P(A \geq 2) = 0.005$, i.e., if the expected number of cases in the study base is 0.100 then the probability of two or more observed cases is 0.005. In the same way one can see that the expected number of cases corresponding to a P-value of 2.5% is 0.242.

The P-value function in the above example is calculated from the Poisson distribution's probability function, and the reason for this is that the Poisson distribution is the probability model best suited to this type of data. The P-value function is in principle obtained in the same way regardless of the type of data; however, the probability model in question does vary from situation to situation, which means that the calculations of probability are performed differently, according to how the probability or frequency function looks. In the rest of this book, exact probability functions will often be approximated with the normal distribution, for which reason an example based on this distribution might be timely here.

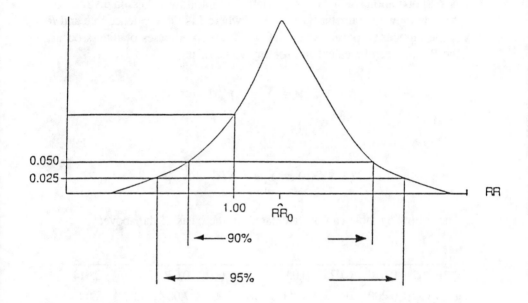

Figure 4.2   The P-value function gives the P-value for all possible values of *RR*, not just *RR* = 1. The "traditional" P-value can be read against *RR* = 1. The P-value function also gives confidence intervals. In the figure, 90 and 95% confidence intervals are marked.

EXAMPLE:

Let us assume that:

$$\hat{\mu} \sim N[\mu, \, var(\hat{\mu})] \quad \text{where} \quad var(\hat{\mu}) = 4.00 \quad \text{and} \quad \hat{\mu}_0 = 2.00$$

The P-value function is then calculated according to:

$$P = \begin{cases} P\left(Z \le \dfrac{2.000 - \mu}{\sqrt{4.00}}\right) & \text{for } \mu > 2.00 \\[3mm] P\left(Z \ge \dfrac{2.000 - \mu}{\sqrt{4.00}}\right) & \text{otherwise} \end{cases}$$

A table for the P-value function can now be calculated:

P	0.001	0.006	0.023	0.025	0.067	...	0.067	0.025	0.023	0.006	0.001
μ	-4.00	-3.00	-2.00	-1.92	-1.00	...	5.00	5.92	6.00	7.00	8.00

This table is interpreted in the same way as that for the Poisson distribution. If, for example, $\mu = 6.00$, then the P-value is 0.023. The two μ-values which correspond to $P = 0.025$ are $\mu = -1.92$ and $\mu = 5.92$. They may be calculated as:

$$\hat{\mu} \pm 1.96 \sqrt{var(\hat{\mu})} = -1.92, 5.92$$

where 1.96 corresponds to the probability 0.025 in the standardized normal distribution.

By looking at the P-value function one can determine which values of the parameter, for example RR, are consistent with the observed study outcome. This gives considerably more information than if one merely calculates the P-value which corresponds to the null hypothesis. This P-value only indicates the degree of consistency between the data and the null hypothesis. The P-value function indicates the degree of consistency with a range of possible parameter values.

It is actually neither practically possible nor necessary to present the whole P-value function. The two values corresponding to $P = 0.025$, for example, give considerable information about the shape and location of the P-value function. In the next section we will see that these two values also constitute the limits for a 95% confidence interval.

4.3 THE CONFIDENCE INTERVAL

4.3.1 What is the Confidence Interval?

By confidence interval we mean an interval constructed according to such a principle that it will, with a certain probability, contain the desired parameter value. If, for example, a study results in a 95% confidence interval for *RR* ranging from 0.900 to 2.50, this means that the interval is calculated according to a principle whereby 95 out of 100 intervals give an interval which contains the true *RR* value. One is 95% "confident" in the assertion that the true value falls within this interval. One might be concerned that the choice of confidence level is as arbitrary as the choice of significance level, which was earlier rejected. However, one should not concentrate on the upper or lower limit but rather on the general position of the interval. The confidence interval can be understood as a summary of the P-value function; the relationship between the P-value function and the confidence interval will be discussed later in this section. If the confidence interval is understood as a description of the P-value function, interest is focused on the general localization of the confidence interval rather than on its two limits, and the choice of confidence level is thus of less importance.

A not uncommon mistake is to look only at the lower limit of the confidence interval. If the estimated parameter is *RR* then the answer to whether the confidence interval's lower limit exceeds or falls below 1.00 can be directly translated into a significant or non-significant test result. However, this is merely a complicated way of carrying out a significance test and is neither better nor worse than one which is performed directly.

Thus, the whole interval should be taken into account when interpreting the confidence interval. If the interval is too broad and includes values which are consistent with no effect as well as ones which are consistent with considerable effect, the study is merely uninformative, i.e., its precision is low. To be able to interpret a study as indicating that exposure has a great effect on the occurrence of illness, only large excess risks must be consistent with the outcome. For an outcome to argue against an effect, the interval must only contain values which lie near the parameter value which corresponds to no effect, unity in the case of *RR*.

4.3.2 The Confidence Interval and the P-value Function

The confidence interval is directly linked to the P-value function. The two parameters which correspond to $P = \alpha/2$ are the limits for a confidence interval with confidence level $1 - \alpha$. The lower value also defines a one-sided confidence interval with confidence level $1 - \alpha/2$; the upper value correspondingly defines a one-sided confidence interval with level $1 - \alpha/2$. (See Figure 4.2.)

The fact that an interval constructed in this way really is a confidence interval with a given confidence level is demonstrated by the following. Let the true parameter value be μ and let $\hat{\mu}$ be an estimator of μ with the observed outcome $\hat{\mu}_0$. The confidence interval's lower limit can now be set as the value μ_L, for which $P(\hat{\mu} \geq \hat{\mu}_0 | \mu_L) = \alpha/2$; that is, μ_L is determined in such a way that the P-value is equal to $\alpha/2$ when it is calculated according to the hypothesis that the theoretical value is μ_L. Let us now assume that $\mu_L = \mu$, i.e., that the confidence interval's lower limit comes at exactly the true value. If the observed value had instead been greater, then μ_L would also have been greater and the confidence interval would have moved up. The true value would accordingly have come below the interval's lower limit. The probability of this is $\alpha/2$, one of the characteristics of the P-value being that the probability of it falling below a certain value is the same as that value, and vice versa, given the null hypothesis. The probability of the confidence interval's lower limit exceeding the true value is thus $\alpha/2$. The confidence interval's upper limit can be established in a similar way. The probability of it falling under the true value is also $\alpha/2$. Accordingly, the probability of the confidence interval including the true parameter value is $1 - \alpha$. (See Figure 4.3.)

This relation between the confidence interval and the P-value function explains why the confidence interval can be seen as a description of the P-value function. It further demonstrates how the confidence interval can be calculated from the P-value function.

4.3.3 Calculating the Confidence Interval

The previous section demonstrated how confidence intervals can be calculated with the help of the P-value function. It also demonstrated how both one-sided and two-sided confidence intervals can be constructed. For the sake of simplicity, we will henceforth assume that confidence intervals are double-sided with the level 95% with 2.5% of the probability mass at each end of the interval; each limit for this type of interval is also the limit for a one-sided 97.5% confidence interval.

We can accordingly construct the confidence interval by looking for the two values of the unknown parameter which correspond to $P = 0.025$.

EXAMPLE:

In a previous example in this chapter we explained how to obtain the P-value function when an observed value of a Poisson variable equals 2. The table for that example shows that the two values which correspond to $P = 0.025$ are 0.242 and 7.22. Accordingly, the limits of the 95% confidence interval for the parameter of the Poisson distribution are these two values.

EXAMPLE:

The same section also contains an example based on the normal distribution. The estimate was 2.00 and the variance 4.00. The confidence interval is: −1.92, 5.92.

When the estimator used can be assumed to be normally distributed, the limits for the 95% confidence interval are calculated as:

$$\mu_{L,U} = \hat{\mu} \pm 1.96\sqrt{var(\hat{\mu})}$$

where $\hat{\mu}$ is an estimator of μ. The constant 1.96 is the value from the standardized normal distribution which corresponds to 2.5% and accordingly sets the confidence level at 95%, and $var(\hat{\mu})$ is the variance for the estimator which is used. This formula will return again and again when calculating confidence intervals with the aid of the normal distribution approximation. The estimator, $\hat{\mu}$, will vary depending on what is to be estimated, and the variance will therefore also vary; the basic principle will, however, always remain the same.

One alternative version of this method is of great importance in epidemiologic applications. As has been mentioned previously, the probability distributions used in epidemiology are often so asymmetrical that the normal distribution is not a good approximation. However, this can be countered by, for example, using the logarithm transformation, since this has the capacity to reduce large values more than small ones; a logarithm transformation thus results in a less asymmetrical distribution.

Logarithm transformations are used by first creating a confidence interval around $\ln \hat{\mu}$, and then exponentiating the limits of this interval. One thus constructs a confidence interval on the logarithmic scale which is then

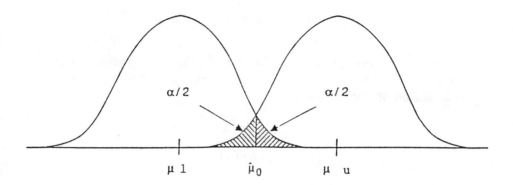

Figure 4.3 The limits for a confidence interval with the level 1 -α obtained as the two parameter values for which the P-value is α/2.

transformed back to the original number scale. A 95% confidence interval according to this principle is therefore constructed as follows:

$$\mu_{L,U} = e^{\ln\hat{\mu} \pm 1.96\sqrt{var(\ln\hat{\mu})}}$$

There are no difficulties in calculating $\ln\hat{\mu}$. How $var(\ln\hat{\mu})$ is calculated depends on each situation. One can often use the variance formula with logarithm transformation (see Section 2.2.3):

$$var(\ln\hat{\mu}) \approx \frac{var(\hat{\mu})}{[E(\hat{\mu})]^2}$$

We will return to this in specific types of situations in later chapters.

An approximate way of calculating confidence intervals which has come to be widely used in epidemiology is the so-called *test-based method*

(Miettinen 1976). If RD is the difference in occurrence of disease between two populations, then an approximate 95% confidence interval can be calculated as follows:

$$\hat{RD} \pm 1.96\sqrt{var(\hat{RD})}$$

In some situations the variance is difficult to estimate. This problem might be countered as follows: To carry out a significance test of the hypothesis, a z value should first be calculated as:

$$z = \frac{\hat{RD}}{\sqrt{var(\hat{RD})}}$$

which would give:

$$\sqrt{var(\hat{RD})} = \frac{\hat{RD}}{z}$$

This expression can be substituted in the formula for the calculation of the confidence interval:

$$\hat{RD} \pm 1.96\frac{\hat{RD}}{z} = \hat{RD}(1 \pm 1.96/z)$$

This means that if one has an estimate of the unknown parameter as well as a z value from a test for that parameter, an approximate confidence interval can be calculated. The advantage here is that the variance of the estimate is not needed; a z value can often be obtained from a conditional test which is carried out without having to estimate the variance of the required parameter.

Test-based confidence intervals can also be calculated for the relative risk. This is usually done by using the logarithm transformation, in which case one gets:

$$e^{\ln \hat{RR}(1 \pm 1.96/z)} = \hat{RR}^{1 \pm 1.96/z}$$

It has been demonstrated that the test-based method gives good results in several types of epidemiologic application, where it is most often used. At the same time it is important to remember that this is an approximate method, which has been criticized from a theoretical standpoint (Gart 1979; Greenland 1984; Halperin 1977).

Confidence intervals which are calculated by approximating the distribution of an estimator with the normal distribution are called *approximate confidence intervals* as opposed to *exact confidence intervals*. Exact confidence intervals are generally complicated to calculate and often necessitate a number of values being successively tested until the probabilities are what they should be (so-called iteration). For this reason, exact intervals are in practice only used when a normal distribution approximation cannot be used, i.e., when the numbers are small.

4.4 PRECISION IN EPIDEMIOLOGIC STUDIES

4.4.1 Evaluating and Reporting the Precision

The purpose of epidemiologic studies is either to estimate the occurrence of disease, by some measurement of incidence or prevalence, or to estimate the effect of exposure on the occurrence of disease, measured as ratios (relative risk) or possibly as the difference in some measure of disease occurrence between the exposed and the non-exposed. Whatever the aim, an observed outcome can diverge from the theoretical value as a result of systematic or random errors. This book concentrates on methods for evaluating random errors and assumes that systematic errors are adequately addressed.

As has been pointed out earlier, significance testing is very commonly used for evaluating random errors in medical research. However, for reasons which should by now be clear, this is an approach which should be avoided.

Even if the thesis proposed above is that the P-value function is the summary of the material which gives the best basis for interpreting it, it is not realistic to present data in the detail which this method demands. One can conclude, therefore, that an appropriate way of reporting on a material is to give a point estimate and a confidence interval. The reason for this is two-fold. Firstly, the confidence interval is a summary of the P-value function; secondly, it also gives an interval of values which, with known confidence, contains the true value.

Attitudes towards the confidence interval have made progress in recent times, and many of the larger journals, for example the *New England Journal of Medicine,* now advocate confidence intervals rather than significance tests. However, this change of opinion has resulted not infrequently in confidence intervals being calculated, only then to be interpreted as if they were significance tests. In other words, the interpretation is entirely based on whether the confidence interval includes the value which corresponds to the exposure having no effect. This is, naturally, no more adequate than the original test procedure.

4.4.2 Analysis of a Multiple Hypotheses

It is usual in epidemiologic studies to be able to analyze a variety of hypotheses at the same time. An example of this is case-control studies which use wide-ranging questionnaires covering such areas as work life, diet, medication, and leisure time activities. It is also the case with studies based on large sets of register material where possible excess risks of, for example, a large number of tumor forms in hundreds of occupational groups can be studied.

It has been suggested that a considerable number of false "significances" are obtained when many analyses are carried out, even if no real effects exist, since the probability of getting a significant result is 5% in each analysis. This has come to be called the *mass significance problem*, or the problem of *multiple comparisons*. The statistical literature offers a variety of methods for compensating for the multiple significance problem (Scheffe 1959; Sverdrup 1976; Sherg 1980; Thomas et al. 1985). Of necessity these result in a conservative interpretation of data, that is, in the requirements for statistical significance being increased. Discussion about the multiple comparison problem arises as a rule in connection with hypothesis testing, but the situation is of course the same when confidence intervals are used.

However, this whole discussion is resolved if the issue is reformulated (Cole 1979; Miettinen 1985; Rothman 1986; Rothman 1989; Rothman 1990). It is, of course, correct that a significance level of 5% will in the long run give significant results in one test in twenty, when no effects are present, and a long series of tests can accordingly be expected to give numerous randomly determined significant findings. However, this lacks relevance unless the null hypothesis is formulated as:

$$RR_1 = RR_2 = ... = RR_K = 1$$

where the *RR*s are relative risks for the various associations, and null hypothesis is rejected when the test outcome for a single one of these *RR* is significant. According to this reasoning it is actually correct that the probability of obtaining significant results increases when the number of analyses increases. It is, however, difficult to imagine a situation in which this null hypothesis is relevant. Instead, a series of single hypotheses about *RR* are tested one at a time, and for each of these, the significance level is the one nominally given, regardless of how many further analyses are carried out.

The multiple comparison problem is often discussed in connection with epidemiologic studies. This is because epidemiologic material, of the type described above, permits the testing of a large number of hypotheses which are entirely without biological or other basis. However, this has nothing to do with the number of possible analyses but rather with the background to the various individual hypotheses.

Each question shall be analyzed separately from the others and independently of the number of other completed or possible analyses. The analysis shall thereby weigh the study's empirical outcomes against the other information from earlier epidemiologic studies, theoretical sources, etc. If the material allows one to analyze the association between, say, eye color and liver cancer, and this type of analysis gives a significant result, then the result is rejected as a random effect. This is not because too many other analyses have been carried out at the same time, but because there is no theoretical basis for the hypothesis. If the material contains data on consumption of fat and colon cancer, the data is interpreted in the same way regardless of how many other associations can be analyzed with the aid of data collected in the same study.

4.4.3 Analysis of Hypotheses not Formulated a Priori

A discussion similar to the one above has been conducted regarding the necessity of formulating hypotheses a priori. It has been claimed that collected data can only be used to test hypotheses formulated in advance. A new hypothesis may be formulated from the material, but this can only be tested in subsequent studies with material collected for that purpose.

However, the deciding factor must be which theoretical basis exists for a hypothesis and not when this basis was produced: a researcher collects material to test hypothesis A and at the same time obtains results which are important for hypothesis B, as yet unknown to him. As long as he does not know about hypothesis B, the result for hypothesis B is interpreted with great caution. However, when the researcher in due course is told about hypothesis B, the result assumes the same importance as the result which was obtained to test hypothesis A.

Chapter 5

DESCRIPTIVE EPIDEMIOLOGIC MEASURES

"I jist want to know how many of yez is deaf, dumb, blind, insane and idiotic — likewise how many convicts there is in the family — what all your ages are, especially the old woman and the young ladies — and how many dollars the old gentleman is worth!"

Saturday Evening Post in 1860. In: Reid-Green KS. The History of Census Tabulation. Scientific American 260:78-83, 1989.

By descriptive epidemiologic measures we here mean measures which describe the occurrence of disease as opposed to those which describe the effect of an exposure on the occurrence of disease. The descriptive epidemiologic measures are incidence rate, cumulative incidence and prevalence. The *incidence rate (I)* is the number of cases of disease in relation to the size of the study base, that is the total time during which the individuals in the study population are at risk of getting the disease; time at risk is usually measured in years. The *cumulative incidence (CI)* is the proportion of individuals in a population getting the disease during a given observation period. The *prevalence (P)*, finally, is the proportion of individuals with a disease in a population at a given point in time. For further discussion of these epidemiologic measures we would refer you to an epidemiology textbook or some of the references given here (Elandt-Johnson 1975; Freeman and Hutchison 1980; Haberman 1978; Hoem 1976).

This chapter explains, for each of the above three measures, how the precision of an observed value, can be determined.

From the statistical point of view, these three epidemiologic measures fall into two groups. The incidence rate has dimensions per time unit (1/time) since the number of cases is related to the time during which individuals are at risk of getting the disease. The cumulative incidence and the prevalence are dimensionless. As a consequence, there is a difference between the probability models, on which the analyses are based, for the incidence rate and those for the cumulative incidence and the prevalence. As a rule, the Poisson distribution is used as the basic model in the first case and the binomial distribution in the second, provided that the rest of the conditions are fulfilled.

5.1 INCIDENCE RATE

Analyses of incidence rate are generally based on the assumption that the number of cases has a Poisson distribution. The total time at risk, summed for all individuals, is understood as an interval of time during which a case of illness could occur at any point in time. A precondition for using this model is that the number of cases is seen as an observation of a stochastic variable while the time at risk is understood as a constant. It is possible to establish probability models where the time at risk is also seen as a stochastic variable. Such models can be used for large materials at least, yet they lead to the same methods as the model used here (Hoem 1987).

Let A be the number of cases and R the time at risk in the study base. We assume that A is Poisson-distributed with the parameter μ, where $\mu = IR$. I is the theoretical incidence rate to be estimated. For the estimation, the observed incidence rate is used:

$$\hat{I} = \frac{A}{R}$$

To obtain a confidence interval for the incidence rate, I, a confidence interval is first established for the Poisson distribution's parameter $\mu = IR$, after which the limits for this interval are divided by R. Two main principles for this will be described here. The first is based on the exact probability function of the Poisson distribution and the other on the approximation of the Poisson distribution with the normal distribution.

5.1.1 Exact Method

The exact method employs the Poisson distribution's probability function discussed in Chapter 2 and the discussion of the confidence interval and the

P-value function from Chapter 4. The 95% confidence interval's two limits, μ_L and μ_U, are obtained by solving the equations:

$$\sum_{i=0}^{A} \frac{e^{-\mu_U} \mu_U^i}{i!} = 0.025$$

and

$$\sum_{i=A}^{\infty} \frac{e^{-\mu_L} \mu_L^i}{i!} = 0.025$$

The equations are solved by iteration, that is, by successively testing various μ-values until their sum on the left side is 0.025. However, as soon as the number of cases rises to, say, 15 to 20, there is no longer any reason to use the exact method, since normal distribution approximations will then give results which, for all practical purposes, are equivalent to results obtained by the exact method.

Since the confidence interval for the Poisson distribution's parameter only depends on the observed number of cases, it is easy to compile a table which gives the confidence interval for different numbers of cases. A table of this kind is to be found in Appendix 1.

EXAMPLE:

Assume that a study gives results of $A = 15$ and $R = 2,000$. The table in Appendix 1 shows that a 95% confidence interval for μ is 8.395, 24.74. The confidence interval for I is obtained by dividing both of these limits by $R = 2,000$. This gives $I_L, I_U = 0.00420, 0.0124$.

5.1.2 Normal Distribution Approximation

A confidence interval based on approximation with the normal distribution assumes that $A \sim N(\mu, \mu)$, where A is used as an estimation of μ (see Chapter 2). A confidence interval for μ is established as follows:

$$\mu_{L, U} = A \pm 1.96\sqrt{A}$$

after which the two limits are divided by R.

NOTE: The variance of the Poisson distribution is the same as its mean value. This means, provided no *variance stabilizing transformation* has been carried out, that the variance varies when the parameter varies. It also means that the variance is different at the two limits of the confidence interval. In the above formula the variance has been set at A, that is, at the value of the mid-point of the confidence interval. An alternative possibility, which would improve the approximation, would be to set the variance as equal to the limit of the confidence interval, so that

$$\mu_L = A - 1.96\sqrt{\mu_L}$$

and

$$\mu_U = A + 1.96\sqrt{\mu_U}$$

The problem with this approach is of course that one has to know the result before one can calculate it! This problem can be solved, but it is only important in the case of small numbers, in which case it is better to use the exact method employing the table in Appendix 1.

The normal distribution approximation enables one to calculate the confidence interval for I directly by regarding A/R as an estimator. Since A is approximately normally distributed and R is a constant, A/R is also approximately normally distributed. The variance is $var(A/R) = var(A)/R^2$ and is estimated as A/R^2.

Thus, an approximate 95% confidence interval for I is obtained as follows:

$$\frac{A}{R} \pm 1.96\sqrt{\frac{A}{R^2}}$$

EXAMPLE:

If, again, $A = 15$ and $R = 2000$, the confidence interval will be:

$$I_{L, U} = \frac{15}{2000} \pm \sqrt{\frac{15}{2000^2}} = 0.00370, 0.0113$$

To get an idea of the reliability of the approximation one can compare it with the corresponding result obtained from the exact calculations.

5.2 CUMULATIVE INCIDENCE

The binomial distribution is generally the starting point for analyzing the cumulative incidence (*CI*). If *A* is the number of cases of disease, then $A \sim bin(n, p)$, where *n* is the size of the population under study and *p* the cumulative incidence.

5.2.1 Exact Method

An exact 95% confidence interval for *CI* is obtained from the equations:

$$\sum_{i=0}^{A} \binom{n}{i} p_U^i (1 - p_U)^{n-i} = 0.025$$

$$\sum_{i=A}^{n} \binom{n}{i} p_L^i (1 - p_L)^{n-i} = 0.025$$

Just as when exact confidence intervals for the incidence rate were calculated using the Poisson distribution, the equations are solved by iteration, whereby different values of *p* are tested until the sum on the left is 0.025. Standard programs for calculating exact confidence intervals for the binomial distribution can be used for this purpose. See also Table 2 in Appendix 1.

5.2.2 Approximations

For large materials the normal distribution approximation is used. Here, A/N is assumed to be approximately normally distributed with $E(A/N) = p = CI$ and $var(A/N) = p (1 - p)/N$ which is estimated as $[A/N(1 - A/N)]/N$. The approximate 95% confidence interval will be:

$$CI_{L, U} = \frac{A}{N} \pm 1.96 \sqrt{\frac{\frac{A}{N} (1 - \frac{A}{N})}{N}}$$

This approximation can be used for reasonably large materials if the binomial distribution is not too asymmetric. The asymmetry is determined by p and will be large with low p-values. It follows that this approximation is only suitable for common diseases.

An alternative approximation process can often be used in epidemiology because of the low frequency of many diseases. Here, one approximates the binomial distribution with the Poisson distribution. The same procedures are used as those for analyzing the incidence rate which were described in the previous section; that is, the limits of the confidence intervals can be determined by using the exact or the approximate method, and when the exact method is applied, Table 1 in Appendix 1 can still be used.

EXAMPLE:

Assume that $A = 5$ cases of disease occur in a population of $N = 10,000$ individuals. The binomial distribution is the basic model and $A \sim bin(10,000, CI)$. The cumulative incidence is low, however, and the Poisson distribution gives a good approximation of the binomial distribution. For this approximation the Poisson distribution's parameter $\mu = 10,000 \times CI$, that is, it is equal to the mean value of the binomial distribution. A 95% confidence interval for μ of 1.623, 11.668 is obtained from the table in Appendix 1. The confidence interval for CI is obtained by dividing these two limits by $N = 10,000$, which gives 0.000162, 0.00117.

5.3 PREVALENCE

The model used for analyzing prevalence is the same as that for the cumulative incidence, i.e., the binomial distribution. The number of individuals who have the disease at a certain point in time is assumed to be $bin(n, p)$, where n is the size of the population and p is the prevalence. The confidence interval is determined in exactly the same way as in Section 5.2.

Chapter 6

MEASURES OF EFFECT FOR CRUDE ANALYSIS

"I have noticed of late," said King Harald, *"that young people cling less keenly to life than old people."*

Bengtsson FG: Röde Orm. P.A. Norstedt & Söners Förlag 1941, 1945.

Measure of effect here means measures which describe the effect on the occurrence of disease of a certain exposure (in epidemiology, the term exposure has a wide meaning and includes such features as genetic factors, socio-economic status, etc.). The most common measures of effect are the difference in disease occurrence between exposed and unexposed and the ratio of disease occurrence between exposed and unexposed. The latter is the most common and will be considered in greatest detail. The ratio between the occurrence of disease among the exposed and the unexposed is usually called the *relative risk* (*RR*); the measure of disease occurrence used is not always a measure of risk in the true sense and *rate ratio* might be a more appropriate notation for the ratio of incidence rates.

The basic measure of occurrence of disease is the incidence rate, which is why the basic measure of effect is either the difference or the ratio between incidence rates. Measures of effect based on the cumulative incidence also have an important function and even measures of effect based on prevalence can give useful information in certain situations. All these options will therefore be taken up here. The *odds-ratio* is used in case-control studies and sometimes with prevalence data; we therefore also describe methods for analyzing odds ratios. For further information, we refer the reader to a textbook on epidemiology.

This chapter looks at *crude data*, that is data which are not *stratified* according to sex, age, smoking, or anything else. We will look at methods for stratified analysis in the next chapter.

6.1 INCIDENCE RATE

The incidence rate is the number of new cases in relation to the total time at risk in the study base. The probability theory model used in analyses of the incidence rate is the Poisson distribution. The use of the Poisson distribution for this purpose was described in the previous chapter in connection with the analysis of descriptive epidemiological measures. The discussion here follows on directly from that in the previous chapter.

The notations used are summarized in the table below:

	Exposure		
	Yes	No	Total
Cases	A_1	A_0	A
Person years	R_1	R_0	R

6.1.1 Difference

Let us first consider the difference between incidence rates. I_1 and I_0 are the incidence rates among exposed and unexposed. Let

$$RD = I_1 - I_0$$

be the measure of effect to be estimated. As previously, the observed incidence rates are used as estimates. One therefore obtains as an estimate of the measure of effect:

$$\hat{RD} = \hat{I}_1 - \hat{I}_0$$

If the study is sufficiently large, this estimate is approximately normally distributed with the mean RD. Since A_1/R_1 and A_0/R_0 are assumed to be independent stochastic variables and since R_1 and R_0 are assumed to be constants, the variance of the estimator is:

$$var(R\hat{D}) = var\left(\frac{A_1}{R_1} - \frac{A_0}{R_0}\right) = var\left(\frac{A_1}{R_1}\right) + var\left(\frac{A_0}{R_0}\right) =$$

$$= \left(\frac{1}{R_1}\right)^2 var(A_1) + \left(\frac{1}{R_0}\right)^2 var(A_0)$$

Both A_1 and A_0 are assumed to be Poisson distributed and the variance is consequently estimated with A_1 and A_0 respectively. We thus get:

$$var(R\hat{D}) \approx \frac{A_1}{R_1^2} + \frac{A_0}{R_0^2} = \frac{\hat{I}_1}{R_1} + \frac{\hat{I}_0}{R_0}$$

An approximate 95% confidence interval for RD can therefore be calculated as:

$$R\hat{D} \pm 1.96 \sqrt{\frac{A_1}{R_1^2} + \frac{A_0}{R_0^2}}$$

in accordance with the principles discussed in Section 4.3.3.

EXAMPLE:

Consider again the example in Section 4.1.2:

	Exposure		
	Yes	No	Total
Cases	25	10	35
Person years	1,000	500	1,500

The confidence interval for the difference between the incidence rates of the two populations is then:

$$RD_{L,U} = \frac{25}{1000} - \frac{10}{500} \pm 1.96 \sqrt{\frac{25}{1000^2} + \frac{10}{500^2}}$$

$$5.000 \times 10^{-3} \pm 1.96 \times 8.062 \times 10^{-3} =$$

$$= -0.0108, \ 0.0208$$

6.1.2 Ratio

6.1.2.1 The Normal Distribution Approximation

Let us now consider a situation in which the relative risk, or rate ratio, defined as $RR = I_1/I_0$, is the measure of effect used. An estimate of the relative risk is obtained as:

$$\hat{RR} = \frac{\hat{I}_1}{\hat{I}_0} = \frac{A_1/R_1}{A_0/R_0}$$

Since this estimator is a ratio which can never be less than zero and has no upper limit, its distribution is asymmetric and not suitable for approximation with the normal distribution. The confidence interval is therefore calculated by means of logarithm transformation, as described in Section 4.3.3. The logarithm of the observed relative risk has a distribution which is more amenable to being approximated with the normal distribution. First, one performs a variable transformation by logarithmizing the observed relative risk, after which a confidence interval is calculated for $\ln RR$. By antilogarithmizing the two limits of the confidence interval for $\ln RR$, one obtains the desired confidence interval for RR.

To calculate the confidence interval, one needs an estimate of the variance of the logarithmized relative risk. Taking the logarithm gives:

$$\ln R\hat{R} = \ln(\frac{\hat{I}_1}{\hat{I}_0}) = \ln\hat{I}_1 - \ln\hat{I}_0 =$$

$$= \ln\frac{A_1}{R_1} - \ln\frac{A_0}{R_0} = \ln A_1 - \ln R_1 - \ln A_0 + \ln R_0$$

Since R_1 and R_0 are constants and since A_1 and A_0 are independent stochastic variables:

$$var(\ln R\hat{R}) = var(\ln A_1) + var(\ln A_0)$$

In the section on variable transformations in Chapter 2 we described how the variance of a logarithmized stochastic variable can be approximated from the variance for the original variable. If the original variable is X, then:

$$var(\ln X) \approx \frac{var(X)}{E(X)^2}$$

Since we are using Poisson distributed variables here, $var(X) = E(X)$; thus, this variance expression can be simplified as:

$$var(\ln X) \approx \frac{1}{E(X)}$$

Since $E(X)$ can be estimated with A_1 and A_0 respectively, then:

$$var(\ln R\hat{R}) \approx \frac{1}{A_1} + \frac{1}{A_0}$$

The approximate 95% confidence interval for $\ln RR$ is consequently:

$$\ln RR_{L, U} = \ln R\hat{R} \pm 1.96 \sqrt{\frac{1}{A_1} + \frac{1}{A_0}}$$

It is, however, not this confidence interval we are looking for, but rather that for RR. This is obtained by antilogarithmizing the two limits given above.

$$RR_{L,U} = e^{\ln R\hat{R} \pm 1.96 \sqrt{\frac{1}{A_1} + \frac{1}{A_0}}}$$

In other words, the two confidence interval limits are obtained as follows:

$$RR_L = e^{\ln RR_L}; \ RR_U = e^{\ln RR_U}$$

EXAMPLE:

With the same example as above we get:

$$\ln RR_{L,\ U} = \ln \frac{25/1000}{10/500} \pm 1.96 \sqrt{\frac{1}{25} + \frac{1}{10}} =$$

$$= 0.2231 \pm 1.96 \times 0.3742 = -0.5102, \ 0.9565$$

The confidence interval for the relative risk RR is obtained as:

$$RR_{L,\ U} = e^{-0.5102,\ 0.9565} = 0.600, \ 2.60$$

6.1.2.2 The Exact Method

Exact confidence intervals are calculated without using the normal distribution approximation. This was described in Chapter 4 in connection with the general discussion of the calculation of confidence intervals. Exact confidence intervals were also described in Chapter 5 in connection with descriptive epidemiological measures. Exact confidence intervals for measure of effect are based on so-called conditional probability distributions (see Chapter 2).

The probability model used to obtain exact confidence intervals for the relative risk, when this is defined as the ratio between the incidence rates for the exposed and the unexposed, is the conditional distribution of the number of exposed cases, given the total number of cases among the exposed and the unexposed together.

When the number of cases among the exposed and the unexposed follows independent Poisson distributions, the number of exposed cases, given the total number of cases, is binomially distributed. The "number parameter" of the binomial distribution (written as n in Chapter 2) is the total number of cases among the exposed and the unexposed together, i.e., $A = A_1 + A_0$. The "probability parameter" of the binomial distribution (written as p in Chapter 2) is the probability that a case will originate from the exposed population; this probability is $I_1R_1/(I_1R_1 + I_0R_0)$. Given that $A_1 + A_0$ cases occur in all, the probability distribution for the number of exposed cases is:

$$A_1 \sim bin\left(A_1 + A_0, \ \frac{I_1R_1}{I_1R_1 + I_0R_0}\right)$$

Exact confidence intervals for the probability parameter in this binomial distribution are calculated by the same methods as for other binomial distributions (see the section on this in Chapter 4 and also that on confidence intervals for cumulative incidence in Chapter 5). The calculations are iterative and standard programs are used to perform them. The confidence limits obtained in this way are transformed into limits for a confidence interval for RR as follows. Let

$$p = \frac{I_1R_1}{I_1R_1 + I_0R_0}$$

By dividing both the numerator and the denominator on the right by I_0, $RR = I_1/I_0$ is introduced into the equation. This is then solved for RR:

$$RR = \frac{R_0p}{R_1(1 - p)}$$

By inserting the two confidence interval limits for p into this expression, the corresponding two limits for RR are obtained.

EXAMPLE:

Let us look at the material in the table:

Number of	Exposure		
	Yes	No	Total
Cases	4	1	5
Person years	1,000	500	1,500

Five cases in all have thus occurred and the number of exposed cases consequently follows a binomial distribution with $n = A_1 + A_0 = 5$. A 95% confidence interval for the probability parameter, p, can be calculated as 0.2836, 0.9950. See Table 2 in Appendix 1. By inserting these limits into the above expression one obtains $RR_{L,U} = 0.198, 99.5$.

6.1.2.3 Test-Based Confidence Intervals

Chapter 4 also dealt with the principles for so-called test-based confidence intervals (see Section 4.3.3). These offer a simple method for calculating approximate confidence intervals. The formula for the test-based confidence interval is:

$$RR_{L, U} = \hat{RR}^{(1 \pm 1.96/z)}$$

Where z is the outcome of a standardized, normally distributed test variable which tests the hypothesis that $RR = 1$. The z-value is often obtained by means of a test which uses the same conditional distribution as the exact analysis, but where the normal distribution approximation instead of the exact probability distribution (see previous section) is used. This avoids the necessity to calculate a variance for the estimator in question.

Under the hypothesis that $RR = 1$, the probability parameter in the conditional binomial distribution in the previous section is $p = R_1/(R_1 + R_0)$.

The binomial distribution's n-parameter is $n = A$. By calculating the mean value and the variance of the binomial distribution and by using these to approximate the binomial distribution with the normal distribution, one obtains:

$$z = \frac{A_1 - A \dfrac{R_1}{R_1 + R_0}}{\sqrt{A \dfrac{R_1}{R_1 + R_0} \left(1 - \dfrac{R_1}{R_1 + R_0}\right)}}$$

EXAMPLE:

Let us again consider the example where there are 25 cases and 1,000 person years among the exposed and 10 cases and 500 person years among the unexposed. To calculate a test-based confidence interval we need an estimate of the relative risk and a value for the test variable, z. The relative risk is calculated in the usual way:

$$\hat{RR} = \frac{25/1000}{10/500} = 1.250$$

The test variable is calculated from the mean value and the variance of the binomial distribution, given the hypothesis that $RR = 1$. We thus get a mean value of:

$$35 \times 1{,}000/1{,}500 = 23.33$$

and a variance of:

$$35 \times 1{,}000/1{,}500 \times (1 - 1{,}000/1{,}500) = 7.778$$

Thus,

$$z = \frac{25 - 23.33}{\sqrt{7.778}} = 0.5988$$

The test-based confidence interval will thus be:

$$RR_{L,U} = 1.250^{(1 \pm 1.96/0.5988)} = 0.602, \ 2.59$$

This result can be compared with that for the example in Section 6.1.2.1.

6.2 CUMULATIVE INCIDENCE

The cumulative incidence is the number who get the disease in relation to the number who are at risk of getting the disease at the beginning of the observation period. The basic probability theory model used for analyzing the cumulative incidence is the binomial distribution. The principles for this have already been described in the previous chapter in connection with the analysis of descriptive epidemiological measures. The discussion of the analysis of measures of effect based on cumulative incidence is a direct continuation of the discussion in the previous chapter.

Just as with measures of effect based on incidence rates, the description we give here will be divided into methods for analyzing difference and those for ratios. With low probabilities, the binomial distribution will be approximately Poisson-distributed. Since cumulative incidences are often low, this is a useful approximation procedure, which will also be discussed.

The notations used are given in the table below:

| Disease | Exposure | | |
	Yes	No	Total
Yes	A_1	A_0	A
No	$N_1 - A_1$	$N_0 - A_0$	$N - A$
Total	N_1	N_0	N

6.2.1 Difference

Let $RD = CI_1 - CI_0$ be the measure of effect to be estimated. This is done by using the corresponding observed value, which is approximately normally distributed in sufficiently large materials. The variance is estimated:

$$var(R\hat{D}) = var(\hat{CI_1}) + var(\hat{CI_0}) \approx \frac{\hat{CI_1}(1 - \hat{CI_1})}{N_1} + \frac{\hat{CI_0}(1 - \hat{CI_0})}{N_0}$$

An approximate 95% confidence interval can now be calculated:

$$RD_{L,U} = R\hat{D} \pm 1.96 \sqrt{\frac{\hat{CI_1}(1 - \hat{CI_1})}{N_1} + \frac{\hat{CI_0}(1 - \hat{CI_0})}{N_0}}$$

EXAMPLE:

Consider the data in the table below:

	Exposure		
Disease	Yes	No	Total
Yes	25	10	35
No	975	490	1,465
Total	1,000	500	1,500

The difference in the cumulative incidence is estimated as $25/1{,}000 - 10/500 = 5.000 \times 10^{-3}$. The variance for this estimate is taken as:

$$var(R\hat{D}) \approx \frac{\frac{25}{1000} \times \frac{975}{1000}}{1000} + \frac{\frac{10}{500} \times \frac{490}{500}}{500} = 6.358 \times 10^{-5}$$

The confidence interval is therefore:

$$CI_{L,U} = 5.000 \times 10^{-3} \pm 1.96\sqrt{6.358 \times 10^{-5}} = -0.0106, 0.0206$$

6.2.2 Ratio

6.2.2.1 Normal Distribution Approximation

As has been shown above, the relative risk can be formed not only as the ratio between incidence rates, but also as the ratio between cumulative incidences. In general, the notation RR is used for the relative risk, irrespective of the underlying measure of disease occurrence; the reason for this is that the dimension is always the same and that the relative risk based on cumulative incidences usually gives a good approximation of the relative risk based on incidence rates. It is of course always necessary to indicate how a relative risk has been defined.

The statistical analysis of a relative risk based on cumulative incidence follows the same pattern as for incidence rates; the important difference is that the basic probability model for cumulative incidence is the binomial distribution. Confidence intervals are first calculated on the logarithmic scale, after which the limits are transformed to the ordinary number scale. We thus get the measure of effect $RR = CI_1/CI_0$ which is estimated:

$$\hat{RR} = \frac{\hat{CI}_1}{\hat{CI}_0} = \frac{A_1/N_1}{A_0/N_0}$$

The logarithm transformation gives:

$$\ln\hat{RR} = \ln\frac{A_1}{N_1} - \ln\frac{A_0}{N_0} = \ln A_1 - \ln N_1 - \ln A_0 + \ln N_0$$

Since the number of new cases among exposed and unexposed is assumed to be independent and since the population sizes, N_1 and N_0, are constants, then:

$$var(\ln\hat{RR}) = var(\ln A_1) + var(\ln A_0)$$

The two variances on the right are calculated by using the fact that A_1 and A_0 are binomially distributed as well as the formula from the section on variable transformations in Chapter 2, which describes how one obtains the variance for a logarithmized variable by means of the original variance. The variance of the binomial distribution gives:

$$var(A_1) \approx N_1 \frac{A_1}{N_1} \left(1 - \frac{A_1}{N_1} \right)$$

and the corresponding for A_0. According to the variance formula for logarithmized variables we get:

$$var(\ln A_1) \approx \frac{var(A_1)}{E(A_1)^2}$$

and the corresponding for A_0. By substituting the variance estimate and an estimate of the mean in this expression for each of the exposed and unexposed groups respectively, one obtains the following estimate of the variance for the logarithmized relative risk:

$$var(\ln R\hat{R}) \approx \frac{N_1 - A_1}{N_1 A_1} + \frac{N_0 - A_0}{N_0 A_0}$$

It is educational to note that when A is small in relation to N, i.e., when $(N - A)/N \approx 1$, this variance expression concurs with the corresponding one for the Poisson distribution which was used for the analysis of incidence rates (i.e., with $1/A_1 + 1/A_0$; see Section 6.1.2.1). We can now calculate a 95% approximate confidence interval:

$$RR_{L,U} = e^{\ln R\hat{R} \pm 1.96\sqrt{var(\ln R\hat{R})}}$$

EXAMPLE:

Let us consider once again the example from the previous section:

$$\ln R\hat{R} = \ln \frac{25/1000}{10/500} = \ln 1.250 = 0.2231$$

The variance estimate is:

$$var(\ln R\hat{R}) \approx \frac{1000 - 25}{1000 \times 25} + \frac{500 - 10}{500 \times 10} = 0.1370$$

The confidence interval will be:

$$RR_{L,U} = e^{0.2231 \pm 1.96 \sqrt{0.1370}} =$$

$$= e^{-0.5024, \ 0.9486} = 0.605, \ 2.58$$

In other words, $RR_{L,U} = 0.605, 2.58$. If one compares this with the corresponding example in the section on incidence rates, the close agreement between the two sets of confidence intervals is demonstrated. This illustrates the fact that the Poisson distribution can be used as an approximation with low incidence.

6.2.2.2 The Exact Method

There is no practical, useful method for calculating exact confidence intervals for the relative risk when it is defined as the ratio between cumulative incidences (Rothman 1986). When the cumulative incidences are low, however, the odds ratio can be used as an approximation of the ratio between the cumulative incidences. In Section 6.4.3 we describe how to calculate exact confidence intervals for odds ratios.

6.2.2.3 Test-Based Confidence Intervals

In this situation too, an approximation can easily be obtained by means of the test-based method. Here, a test variable, z, must be calculated from the conditional probability distribution for the number of exposed cases. The number of cases among the exposed and the unexposed are assumed to be independently binomially distributed variables. The number of exposed cases, conditional upon the total number of cases, is thus hypergeometrically distributed, on the condition that $RR = 1$. The test variable, z, is calculated as:

$$z = \frac{A_1 - E(A_1)}{\sqrt{var(A_1)}}$$

where

$$E(A_1) = A\,\frac{N_1}{N}$$

and where

$$var(A_1) = \frac{A(N - A)N_1 N_0}{N^2(N - 1)}$$

Just as before, the approximate 95% confidence interval is:

$$RR_{L,U} = R\hat{R}^{(1 \pm 1.96/z)}$$

EXAMPLE:

With the same data as in the previous example we get:

$$A_1 = 25;\ E(A_1) = 35\,\frac{1,000}{1,500} = 23.33$$

$$var(A_1) = \frac{35 \times 1,465 \times 1,000 \times 500}{1,500^2 \times (1,500 - 1)} = 7.596$$

$$z = \frac{25 - 23.33}{\sqrt{7.596}} = 0.6059$$

The confidence interval will be:

$$RR_{L,U} = 1.250^{(1 \pm 1.96/0.6059)} = 0.607, \ 2.57$$

Again, the results of the different methods can be compared.

6.3 PREVALENCE

Just like the cumulative incidence, the prevalence is a proportion and the basic probability theory model will therefore be the same for analyses of prevalence as for analyses of cumulative incidence. The methods described in previous sections can therefore be directly applied to analyses of relative risks based on prevalence.

In certain situations prevalence is used for practical reasons even though the aim is to estimate a ratio between incidence rates. In such instances one will achieve a better relative risk estimate if a prevalence-odds ratio is calculated; this is especially the case with common diseases. In such situations, the analysis of the data does not follow the lines discussed above but rather the methods which are taken up in the following section.

6.4 ODDS RATIOS

6.4.1 Relative Risk, Odds Ratios, and Case-Control Studies

The purpose of a case-control study is to estimate the relative risk, (usually) defined as the ratio between the incidence rate for the exposed and the unexposed. (See one of the textbooks on epidemiology in the reference list). The estimate of the relative risk which was used in Section 6.1.2 can be rewritten as:

$$\hat{RR} = \frac{A_1/R_1}{A_0/R_0} = \frac{A_1/A_0}{R_1/R_0}$$

The numerator on the far right is the ratio between the number of exposed and unexposed cases and the denominator is the ratio between the number of exposed and unexposed person years. An odds ratio is the ratio between the number in a particular category and the remainder. Both the numerator and the denominator on the far right are odds and the ratio is consequently an *odds ratio*. The estimate of the relative risk can thus be written in such a way that it can be called, in mathematical terms, an odds ratio.

By *case-control study* we mean a study where a sample from the study base is used to estimate R_1/R_0. This sample is the case-control study's control group. The material in a case-control study can accordingly be said to be comprised of a series of cases distributed between exposed and unexposed and a series of controls distributed in the same way. The relative risk is estimated by means of the odds ratio. The notations in the table below are often used for case-control studies; the table is also the easiest way of presenting the material:

	Exposure		
	Yes	No	Total
Cases	a	b	N_1
Controls	c	d	N_0
Total	M_1	M_0	T

This simple fourfold table has attracted great interest among biostatisticians and much has been written on various attempts at analysis (see, for example, Breslow and Day 1980). Here we can only give an idea of the extensive literature which exists on the subject.

The following odds ratio is used as an estimate of the relative risk:

$$\hat{OR} = \frac{a/b}{c/d} = \frac{ad}{bc}$$

For the statistical analysis, the number of exposed cases and the number of exposed controls are assumed to be independent, binomially distributed variables with the parameters N_1, p_1, N_0 and p_0, where p_1 and p_0 are the probabilities of exposure among cases and among controls; the purpose of the analysis is to establish a confidence interval for the odds ratio:

$$OR = \frac{p_1/(1 - p_1)}{p_0/(1 - p_0)}$$

which is thus the parameter in this statistical model which corresponds to the relative risk.

NOTE: It will be clear from the above that the measure of effect used for case-control studies is the same as for cohort studies, that is, the relative risk. The fact that odds ratios are used in case-control studies is not because the effect is measured in a different way but rather because the relative risk is estimated by means of odds-ratios since the exposure distribution in the study base is estimated from a random sample.

6.4.2 Normal Distribution Approximation

In the main, the statistical analysis for the normal distribution approximation follows the same principles as in the previous sections of this chapter. The estimator is:

$$\hat{OR} = \frac{ad}{bc}$$

For the same reasons as before, one must first establish the confidence interval on the logarithmic scale, after which the limits of this interval are antilogarithmized.

Since $b = N_1 - a$ and $d = N_0 - c$, we write:

$$\ln\hat{OR} = \ln \frac{a}{N_1 - a} - \ln \frac{c}{N_0 - c}$$

which is assumed to be approximately normally distributed, with the variance:

$$var(\ln\hat{OR}) \approx \frac{1}{a} + \frac{1}{b} + \frac{1}{c} + \frac{1}{d}$$

The variance is obtained by means of the same approximation formula as was previously used for logarithmized transformations (see Section 2.2.3).

NOTE: The two last terms in the previous equation for the variance refer to the contribution of the control group to the random uncertainty. When c and d

increase these two terms move towards zero and the remainder becomes $1/a + 1/b$. Note that this is the same equation for variance as that used in the analysis of incidence rates in Section 6.1.2.1. This illustrates the fact that when the control group in a case-control study increases, the case-control study moves closer to the corresponding cohort study.

Thus, an approximate 95% confidence interval for the relative risk in a case control study can be calculated as follows (Woolf 1955):

$$OR_{L, U} = e^{\ln\frac{ad}{bc} \pm 1.96\sqrt{\frac{1}{a} + \frac{1}{b} + \frac{1}{c} + \frac{1}{d}}}$$

EXAMPLE:

Let us assume that a case-control study has given the following data:

	Exposure		
	Yes	No	Total
Cases	100	50	150
Controls	100	100	200
Total	200	150	350

The following can then be calculated:

$$\hat{OR} = \frac{100 \times 100}{100 \times 50} = 2.000 \quad \text{and} \quad \ln\hat{OR} = 0.6931$$

and

$$var(\ln\hat{OR}) \approx \frac{1}{100} + \frac{1}{50} + \frac{1}{100} + \frac{1}{100} = 0.05000$$

Thus, the 95% confidence interval is:

$$OR_{L,U} = e^{0.6931 \pm 1.96\sqrt{0.0500}} =$$

$$= e^{0.6931 \pm 0.4383} = e^{0.2549, \ 1.131} = 1.29, \ 3.10$$

NOTE: In Chapter 5 we discussed the problem that the variance for the estimate can vary according to the parameter value and that it is not entirely correct to use, at the limits of a confidence interval, a variance which is based on the mid-point of the interval. Cornfield (1956) has suggested a method for case-control study data based on the normal distribution approximation which takes this into account. A more general method has also been suggested (Miettinen 1985; Miettinen and Nurminen 1985).

6.4.3 Exact Method

For the type of data we are discussing here, the exact method is based on the conditional probability distribution for the number of exposed cases given the total number of exposed. It is worth noting that since the number of cases and the number of controls are known from the start, all margin sums are fixed as soon as the total number of exposed is given. It thus follows that just one of the four cells a, b, c and d determines the other three.

When the numbers of exposed among the cases and controls follow two independent binomial distributions, the conditional numbers of exposed cases are distributed according to the non-central hypergeometrical distribution (see Section 2.3.4). This distribution has, with the notations we use here, the probability function:

$$p(a) = \frac{\binom{N_1}{a}\binom{N_0}{M_1-a}OR^a}{\sum_i \binom{N_1}{i}\binom{N_0}{M_1-i}OR^i}$$

When $OR = 1$ this simplifies to the usual hypergeometrical distribution, since the OR − expressions cancel out and since:

$$\sum_i \binom{N_1}{i}\binom{N_0}{M_1-i} = \binom{N_1+N_0}{M_1}$$

This is used to calculate the P-value on the assumption that the null hypothesis is correct. To calculate the exact 95% confidence interval one uses the probability distribution with the non-central hypergeometrical distribution:

the P-value function is calculated from the observed number of exposed cases and set at 0.025, in order to obtain the confidence level 95%. The confidence interval for OR is established iteratively by successively testing various OR values until the correct probabilities, that is 0.025, are obtained for the lower and for the upper limit. A great many calculations must be carried out for each iteration and a large number of iterations can be necessary. One therefore needs a program for such calculations.

EXAMPLE:

Assume that the study in the previous example was only one tenth the size:

	Exposure		
	Yes	No	Total
Cases	10	5	15
Controls	10	10	20
Total	20	15	35

The estimate will still be 2.000, since:

$$\hat{OR} = \frac{10 \times 10}{10 \times 5} = 2.000$$

The exact 95% confidence limits can be calculated as:

$$OR_{L,U} = 0.414, \ 10.2$$

To study the appropriateness of the normal approximation it can be of interest also to calculate the confidence interval by Woolf's method, which was described in the previous section. With this method, the 95% confidence interval is:

$$OR_{L,U} = 0.500, \ 8.00$$

6.4.4 Test-Based Confidence Interval

Approximate confidence intervals for data from case control studies can also be calculated by the test-based method. The formula for this is, just as before:

$$OR_{L,U} = \hat{OR}^{1 \pm 1.96/z}$$

where the odds ratio is calculated in the same way as above and where 1.96 specifies the 95% confidence level. The test variable z should derive from a test of the hypothesis that $OR = 1$. By basing this test on the same conditional distribution that was used for calculating the exact confidence interval one avoids the need to estimate the variance of the point estimate (or its logarithm).

Let us once again look at the table giving the basic material of a case-control study:

	Exposure		
	Yes	No	Total
Cases	a	b	N_1
Controls	c	d	N_0
Total	M_1	M_0	T

As was mentioned previously, the conditional probabilities (given the total number of exposed M_1) follow the hypergeometrical distribution under the assumption that $OR = 1$. A test can therefore be based on this distribution. However, the aim is to achieve a method for calculating confidence intervals which can be used with large materials. For this reason, the hypergeometrical distribution is approximated with the normal distribution. The mean value and the variance of the hypergeometrical distribution are needed for this:

$$E(a) = \frac{M_1 N_1}{T}$$

$$var(a) = \frac{M_1 M_0 N_1 N_0}{T^2(T-1)}$$

The test variable needed for the confidence interval is calculated as:

$$z = \frac{a - E(a)}{\sqrt{var(a)}}$$

EXAMPLE:

The data from the example in the section on the normal distribution approximation gives here:

$$a = 100 \quad E(a) = \frac{200 \times 150}{350} = 85.71$$

and

$$var(a) = \frac{200 \times 150 \times 150 \times 200}{350^2 \times (350 - 1)} = 20.99$$

So:

$$z = \frac{100 - 85.71}{\sqrt{20.99}} = 3.118$$

The confidence interval is thus:

$$OR_{L,U} = 2.000^{(1 \pm 1.96/3.118)} = 1.29, 3.09$$

Again, the results of the different methods may be compared.

Chapter 7

MEASURES OF EFFECT IN STRATIFIED ANALYSIS

"Aristotle believed that matter was continuous, that is, one could divide a piece of matter into smaller and smaller bits without any limit: one never came up against a grain of matter that could not be divided further."

Hawking SW: A Brief History of Time. From the Big Bang to Black Holes. Bantam Books 1988.

7.1 PURPOSE AND GENERAL PRINCIPLES

By *stratification* in connection with the analysis of data we mean that a material is divided up into *strata*, according to one or more variables other than exposure and disease. Stratification can also be performed when selecting individuals for a study. The individuals are then distributed over a number of strata in a way that has been determined in advance. However, by stratification we mean here, stratification in connection with the analysis of data.

7.1.1 Confounding and Effect Modification

Stratification is performed for two completely different reasons: to evaluate and possibly control for *confounding* by the stratification variable or, to analyze *effect modification* by the stratification variable. These two concepts are often confused but are entirely different (Miettinen 1974). Confounding is a systematic error (or bias) which may or may not be present in a particular study, while effect modification is connected with how different factors interact to cause disease. A detailed discussion of the concepts of confounding and effect modification would be beyond the scope of this book, however, a brief description should be of value for what follows:

> By confounding we mean that some risk factor, apart from the exposure under study, is distributed differently among exposed and unexposed. One consequence of not controlling for this is that exposed and unexposed would differ in disease occurrence independently of any possible effect the studied exposure may have. In each stratum the stratification variable assumes the same value for both exposed and unexposed. Each stratum-specific estimate is therefore free from confounding by the stratification variable, at least within the limits of the chosen categories for stratification.

EXAMPLE:

> If the exposed group contains more men than women, this will lead to a difference in the incidence of myocardial infarction even if the studied exposure does not have an effect. (The incidence of myocardial infarction is higher for men than for women.) If exposure increases morbidity then the differences in gender distribution causes the effect to be strengthened and the result is a combination of the effect of the studied exposure and the effect of being a man. In this example, gender is a confounder. However, this can be controlled for by stratification by gender. This involves the effect of the exposure being estimated separately for men and women. Both of these stratum-specific estimates are free from confounding by gender.

By effect modification we mean that the effect of the exposure differs between the different strata.

EXAMPLE:

> If the relative risk for a particular exposure and myocardial infarction is 2.0 for men and 4.0 for women then an effect modification of gender is present.

In the stratified analysis of data the effect can be estimated separately for single strata and the effect modification can accordingly be studied by comparing strata.

Effect modification depends on how the effect of the exposure is measured. Effect modification can be present in a particular situation if the effect is measured as the ratio between two incidence rates but be absent if the effect is measured as the difference between the incidence rates, and vice versa. Effect modification is consequently a concept which is rather of a statistical interest. If one wants to indicate that one variable influences the effect of another one, in a biological sense, the terms *synergism* and *antagonism* are used instead (Rothman et al. 1980). The concept *interaction* is used alternatively in the meaning of effect modification and synergism as they have been defined above and we will avoid it in this presentation.

EXAMPLE:

Let us assume that the incidence rates for unexposed women and men are 1.0 and 2.0 per 1,000 person years and 2.0 and 4.0 for the exposed. The relative risk for both men and women is then 2.0 and no effect modification is present. If, on the other hand, the effect is measured as the difference in incidence rates, these will be 1.0 per 1,000 person years for women and 2.0 per 1,000 person years for men; when the effect is measured in this way gender is thus an effect modifier.

This chapter will now describe how stratification can be used to control for confounding. We will look at instances both with and without effect modification. Analysis of synergism and effect modification will be discussed separately in Chapter 12.

7.1.2 Estimating a Uniform Effect Versus Standardization

When data are stratified in order to control for confounding there are, in principle, two conceivable outcomes. The first is that no effect modification by the stratification variable is present. Each stratum specific estimate of the effect is thus an estimate of one and the same value, i.e., of an effect which is the same over all strata. The purpose of the analysis is to use the information from the various strata in the best way for estimating the uniform effect.

The other possible outcome is that effect modification is present. In this case, there is no common effect to be estimated. One possible course of action is then to look at the stratum specific values or some function which describes how the effect varies over strata. One could also carry out a weighing of the stratum specific estimates, even though the effect is different in different strata. The latter procedure is often used, especially in descriptive contexts, when large amounts of data are to be analyzed. However, it is inevitable that the result obtained depends on how the weighing is performed, i.e., on which weights are chosen. A weighing of this type is called *standardization*. Methods for estimating a uniform effect and standardization will be discussed separately in the following two sections.

7.2 ESTIMATING A UNIFORM EFFECT

7.2.1 General Principles

With analyses of nonstratified data there is seldom any doubt about how the estimation should be done — the underlying theoretical value is estimated with the corresponding observed value. When information from different strata is combined to give a common estimate, however, there are various possibilities. One of these is to calculate a simple mean for the stratum specific estimates. A more attractive alternative is to give greater weight to strata with greater precision, but the question is then how this is to be done. We will first discuss generally three principles for how this can be done and then how these principles can be specifically applied to different types of epidemiological data.

7.2.1.1 The Maximum Likelihood Method

The *maximum likelihood method,* or *ML-method,* is a general statistical method for estimation. Here, one chooses as estimate the parameter value which has the "maximum likelihood" for the observed outcome. According to general statistical theories, the ML-method gives estimates which have good statistical properties: ML-estimates have in general the smallest possible variance, which means that the material is used in such a way as to obtain the greatest possible precision. ML-estimates are therefore said to be, in statistical terms, *effective*. Furthermore, ML-estimates have, as a rule, a mean which coincides asymptotically with the estimated parameter value. This means that if the size of the study could be increased beyond all the limits the ML-estimate would be the same as the parameter value. The ML-estimates are said to be *consistent*. Finally, when the materials are sufficiently large, ML-estimates are approximately normally distributed. These qualities mean that one generally aims to use maximum likelihood estimates. For a discussion of the maximum likelihood method we refer the reader to, for example, Breslow and Day (1980).

EXAMPLE:

A simple example of an ML-estimate is the estimation of the incidence rate when the number of cases, A, and the number of person years, R, are known. Just as before, A is presumed to be Poisson distributed with the parameter $I \times R$, where I is the underlying, theoretical incidence rate to be estimated. The so-called *likelihood function*, i.e., the likelihood of the observed outcome, is:

$$L(I) = \frac{e^{-IR}(IR)^A}{A!}$$

$L(I)$ is a function which depends on I, i.e., the parameter to be estimated. The ML-estimate of I is the value for which $L(I)$ assumes its maximum value. Usually, a likelihood function is maximized by establishing the maximum of its logarithm, which often is simpler; $L(I)$ and $\ln L(I)$ have maximum for the same value of I. To find the maximum of the likelihood function in this example, $L(I)$ is first logarithmized, which gives:

$$\ln L(I) = -IR + A \ln IR + \text{constant}$$

The third term is constant in the sense that it is not dependent on I. To maximize this expression, the derivative with respect to I is taken and the so obtained expression is set equal to 0. This equation is solved for I:

$$\frac{d\ln L(I)}{dI} = -R + \frac{AR}{IR} + 0 = 0$$

This gives an ML-estimator of I:

$$\hat{I}_{ML} = \frac{A}{R}$$

That is, the number of cases divided by the number of person years at risk. This estimate is consequently the same as the one used in Chapter 5, where, however, we did not refer to the ML-method. For simple situations such as this, the intuitively reasonable estimator agrees usually with the ML-estimator. In the situations which we look at in this chapter, the mathematics is more complicated and the maximization of the likelihood equation obliges one to use iterative methods (see below).

The maximum likelihood method also offers a principle for estimating the variance; the second derivative is taken of $\ln L(I)$ and the expression thereby obtained is inverted and multiplied by -1. One substitutes the ML-estimate in the resulting expression, whereby the variance of the estimate is obtained:

$$\frac{d}{dI}\left(-R + \frac{A}{I}\right) = -\frac{A}{I^2}$$

By inverting, changing symbols and substituting A/R for I, one obtains:

$$var(\hat{I}_{ML}) \approx \frac{A}{R^2} = \frac{\hat{I}}{R}$$

This estimate also agrees with the one presented in Chapter 5.

The way in which one achieves an estimate using the maximum likelihood method varies according to the situation. An iterative method is necessary when estimating a common effect for stratified data. In other words, a starting value is first calculated which then forms the basis for calculating a further value, which in turn is used for further calculations, and so on, until a new value is sufficiently like its predecessor for one to be able to stop the process. These iterative procedures make the calculations complicated and difficult to perform. One advantage is that this method does not require large numbers in individual strata.

The iterations can be carried out in various ways. For many specific situations, including the ones discussed in this chapter, one can establish special algorithms to perform the iterations. The ML-estimate can, however, also be obtained by using one of the *multivariate methods* (see Chapter 12); this means that the ML-estimate and corresponding variance can be obtained by using one of the general computer programs used for multivariate analyses. Programs of this kind are now also available for personal computers. We will discuss this further in Chapter 12.

For a detailed discussion of specific algorithms for maximum likelihood estimates for stratified epidemiological material we refer the reader to Rothman (1986).

7.2.1.2 Pooling

Pooling is a weighing together of the stratum-specific estimates which approximately minimizes the variance of the estimator; the weights are chosen in proportion to the inverted value of the variance for each stratum specific estimate. If these variances were known, the method would agree with the maximum likelihood method; however, the variances are not known and must be estimated. This means that the method can only be used when each stratum is big enough to provide a stable variance estimate.

Let us, to start with, consider a situation in which the effect is measured by the difference in the occurrence of disease between exposed and unexposed. Using the same symbols as before with the addition of an index i to mark the stratum in question, one obtains a pooled estimate as:

$$\hat{RD}_{pool} = \frac{\sum \frac{1}{var(\hat{RD}_i)} \hat{RD}_i}{\sum \frac{1}{var(\hat{RD}_i)}}$$

The division is carried out to guarantee that the sum of the weights is 1. The variance for this estimate can be estimated by repeated used of the variance formulae for linear combinations, provided that the weights are understood as constants (see Section 2.2.3):

$$var(\hat{RD}_{pool}) = \frac{\sum \left[\frac{1}{var(\hat{RD}_i)} \right]^2 var(\hat{RD}_i)}{\left[\sum \frac{1}{var(\hat{RD}_i)} \right]^2} =$$

$$= \frac{1}{\sum \frac{1}{var(\hat{RD}_i)}}$$

From the estimate and its variance a confidence interval can be calculated on the assumption that the estimate is approximately normally distributed. This assumption is reasonable with sufficiently large materials. The 95% confidence interval will be (see Section 4.3.3):

$$RD_{L,U} = R\hat{D}_{pool} \pm 1.96\sqrt{var(R\hat{D}_{pool})}$$

Now let the measure of effect be the relative risk RR. Pooling is often used here, together with logarithm transformation (again, see Section 4.3.3), the confidence interval will be:

$$RR_{L,U} = e^{\ln R\hat{R}_{pool} \pm 1.96\sqrt{var(\ln R\hat{R}_{pool})}}$$

This principle can be used with all the different types of data which were discussed in the previous chapter. The stratum specific estimate and its variance will, however, vary in form depending on the situation in question. In principle, the results for non-stratified data (Chapter 6) are used in each stratum together with the formulae described above. In the following sections we will describe the specific uses for each of the situations in question.

7.2.1.3 The Mantel-Haenszel Method

The third method for obtaining a combined estimate is the *Mantel-Haenszel estimator*, not to be confused with the *Mantel-Haenszel test*; these were both originally presented in the same article (Mantel-Haenszel 1959). The Mantel-Haenszel estimate was intended for use with data from case-control studies but analogues for cohort studies have also been obtained (Rothman & Boice 1982; Tarone 1981).

Using the same symbols as before, but with the addition of the subscript i to indicate the stratum in question, the Mantel-Haenszel estimator for the case-control study is:

$$\hat{OR}_{MH} = \frac{\sum a_i d_i / T_i}{\sum b_i c_i / T_i}$$

Note the similarity to the corresponding estimator for non-stratified data. This expression can, just like the pooled estimate, be written as a weighted mean, yet using different weights:

$$\hat{OR}_{MH} = \frac{\sum w_i \hat{OR}_i}{\sum w_i} \quad \text{with} \quad w_i = \frac{b_i c_i}{T_i}$$

The weights are proportional to the size of the stratum (divided by bc/T) and are accordingly also at least approximately proportional to the precision of the stratum-specific estimate. The Mantel-Haenszel estimator is a weighing procedure which, when it was presented, was based largely on intuitive qualities. Statistical analyses have since shown that under the null hypothesis the weights are proportional to the inverted variance; that is, the Mantel-Haenszel estimate is optimal under this condition. And analyses have shown that this method generally has good statistical properties (Breslow & Liang 1982). Unlike the pooling discussed above, this method does not need large numbers in each individual stratum; it can actually be used even if each stratum consists of only one case and one control (see the note below about matched case-control studies). Furthermore, the calculations performed when using this method are uncomplicated, in part because no iterations are necessary.

The confidence interval for the Mantel-Haenszel estimate can be determined by using the test-based method. The test variable is obtained in this case by the Mantel-Haenszel test. This is a direct development of the test which was described in connection with test-based confidence intervals in Chapter 6. The observed number of exposed cases, together with their mean and variance, given the total number of cases as well as the distribution across exposed and unexposed of the number of cases and controls together, are calculated separately for each stratum and are then added together across all strata. As with the results for non-stratified data, it is the case that the total number of exposed cases is approximately normally distributed with materials that are sufficiently large. Using the same symbols as before:

$$z = \frac{\sum a_i - \sum M_{1i} N_{1i}/T_i}{\sqrt{\sum \frac{N_{1i} N_{0i} M_{1i} M_{0i}}{T_i^2 (T_i - 1)}}}$$

NOTE: If z is squared, a variable is obtained which under the null-hypothesis is *chi-square distributed* with 1 *degree of freedom* and can be used for a chi-square test. This test differs from other chi-square tests of stratified data in only having one degree of freedom. The Mantel-Haenszel test has the advantage of being particularly sensitive when several strata all indicate that there is an excess risk in one and the same direction. In other types of chi-square tests for this type of data, the difference between the observed and the expected number of cases is squared before totalling. For this reason, the direction of the differences between the observed and the expected number cannot be taken into account. A test of this type can give a significant result even if the differences between the observed and the expected number go in different directions in different strata. Another important characteristic of the Mantel-Haenszel test is that it does not require large numbers in each individual stratum, only when they have been added together over all strata. Also the Mantel-Haenszel test can be used even when each stratum contains only one case and one control.

With the aid of the above estimate and test variable a 95% test-based confidence interval is obtained, as before, by:

$$OR_{MH,L,U} = \hat{OR}_{MH}^{(1 \pm 1.96/z)}$$

For a long time there was no suitable variance estimator available for the Mantel-Haenszel estimator and the confidence interval was then determined mainly by the test-based method. However, a method does now exist, and the confidence interval can therefore also be established in the usual way (Greenland & Robins 1985; Robins et al. 1986). Since the Mantel-Haenszel method estimates the relative risk, logarithm transformation is used as usual to obtain a better approximation of the normal distribution. The variance estimate takes different forms depending on the type of data in question. These forms will be presented in the next section, together with other specifications.

7.2.1.4 Exact Confidence Intervals

In the previous chapter about the analysis of non-stratified data, we also described exact methods for determining confidence intervals. Such methods are also available for stratified material. However, these are complex and are not widely used. We refer the reader to Rothman (1986) for a description of these methods.

7.2.1.5 Applications

The methods described above require the underlying measure of effect to be the same for all strata — in other words, that there is no effect modification. This must consequently be evaluated before the information from the different strata are combined to form a common estimate. Unlike the situation when the P-value was described (Section 4.1.3), this is one where a decision really must be reached, i.e., whether or not the information from individual strata is to be combined to give a single estimate. It is thus reasonable to imagine that this evaluation is based on a statistical test of whether the stratum-specific values are the same or not (Zelen 1971; Mantel et al. 1977). As a rule, however, the number of individuals in each single stratum is so few that the ability of this kind of test to reveal the occurrence of an effect modification is limited. This means that the decision about whether to estimate a uniform effect will be a highly pragmatic one. In practice, data is combined to give a common effect if there are no strong reasons for not doing so. Such reasons can either be the pattern which the stratum-specific estimates demonstrate or subject matter knowledge. Above all, when multivariate methods are used, statistical tests are also used in order to decide whether the effect can be regarded as constant across strata. (See also Chapter 12.)

In the next section we will describe how the principles presented above are applied in the common epidemiologic situations. The greatest difference between these various situations is the difference in the variance expression. In other respects, more or less the same procedures will be repeated time and again.

7.2.2 Incidence Rate

With the same symbols as before and with an index i to indicate the stratum in question, the symbols for data with cases of disease and person years at risk are:

	Exposure		
	Yes	No	Total
Cases	A_{1i}	A_{0i}	A_i
Person years	R_{1i}	R_{0i}	R_i

Let us begin with pooling. The results from Chapter 6 can be applied to each stratum. For stratum i the difference between two incidence rates is therefore estimated as:

$$\hat{RD}_i = \hat{I}_{1i} - \hat{I}_{0i}$$

This estimator has a variance which, for sufficiently large materials, can be taken as (see Section 6.1.1):

$$var(\hat{RD}_i) \approx \frac{A_{1i}}{R_{1i}^2} + \frac{A_{0i}}{R_{0i}^2}$$

The pooled estimate is calculated in the ways described in the last section. The estimator will be:

$$\hat{RD}_{pool} = \frac{\sum \dfrac{1}{\dfrac{A_{1i}}{R_{1i}^2} + \dfrac{A_{0i}}{R_{0i}^2}} \hat{RD}_i}{\sum \dfrac{1}{\dfrac{A_{1i}}{R_{1i}^2} + \dfrac{A_{0i}}{R_{0i}^2}}}$$

Also in accordance with the results in the above section, its variance can be estimated as:

$$var(\hat{RD}_{pool}) \approx \frac{1}{\sum \dfrac{1}{\dfrac{A_{1i}}{R_{1i}^2} + \dfrac{A_{0i}}{R_{0i}^2}}}$$

An approximate 95% confidence interval is calculated by substituting the estimate and its variance in the formula:

$$RD_{pool,L,U} = \hat{RD}_{pool} \pm 1.96\sqrt{var(\hat{RD}_{pool})}$$

To analyze the ratio between two incidence rates one calculates the relative risk in stratum i:

$$\hat{RR}_i = \frac{\hat{I}_{1i}}{\hat{I}_{0i}}$$

Just as before with the normal approximation of relative risks, the logarithm transformation is used. The variance for the logarithm of the above estimator is (see Section 6.1.2):

$$var(\ln\hat{RR}_i) \approx \frac{1}{A_{1i}} + \frac{1}{A_{0i}}$$

The pooled estimator is obtained by pooling the logarithms of the stratum-specific estimators with weights proportional to the inverted variances. An estimator of RR is then obtained by exponentiating. The pooled estimator is thus:

$$\hat{RR}_{pool} = \exp\left[\frac{\sum \frac{1}{\frac{1}{A_{1i}} + \frac{1}{A_{0i}}}\ln\hat{RR}_i}{\sum \frac{1}{\frac{1}{A_{1i}} + \frac{1}{A_{0i}}}}\right]$$

Since the confidence interval is calculated on the logarithmized scale one needs the variance for the logarithm of the RR-estimate. This, again, is the inverted value of the denominator in the estimate:

$$var(\ln\hat{RR}_{pool}) \approx \frac{1}{\sum \frac{1}{\frac{1}{A_{1i}} + \frac{1}{A_{0i}}}}$$

An approximate 95% confidence interval is calculated, as before, by using the normal distribution approximation on the logarithmized scale, after which the limits are antilogarithmized to the original number scale:

$$RR_{pool,L,U} = \exp[\ln R\hat{R}_{pool} \pm 1.96 \sqrt{var(\ln R\hat{R}_{pool})}\ ]$$

Let us now continue with the Mantel-Haenszel method. As was mentioned earlier, the original version of the Mantel-Haenszel estimator was for data from case-control studies (Mantel-Haenszel 1959). A version for incidence rates was, however, presented later (Rothman and Boice 1982). Using the same symbols as above, this estimator is:

$$R\hat{R}_{MH} = \frac{\sum A_{1i} R_{0i}/R_i}{\sum A_{0i} R_{1i}/R_i}$$

An approximate 95% confidence interval can be simply established as follows, by means of the test-based method:

$$RR_{MH,L,U} = R\hat{R}_{MH}^{(1 \pm 1.96/z)}$$

The necessary z-value is calculated by means of a version of the Mantel-Haenszel test, adapted for data with incidence rates. This version uses the method for calculating a test variable for incidence rate data based on the binomial distribution, (see Section 6.2.3.4), as well as the method by which one adds together across strata, taken from the original Mantel-Haenszel test (see Section 7.2.1.3):

$$A_1 = \sum A_{1i}, \ E(A_1) = \sum A_i \frac{R_{1i}}{R_i}$$

and

$$var(A_1) = \sum A_i \frac{R_{1i}}{R_i}\left(1 - \frac{R_{1i}}{R_i}\right)$$

Just as before, the z-value is obtained as:

$$z = \frac{A_1 - E(A_1)}{\sqrt{var(A_1)}}$$

The value for z obtained in this way is used to determine the test-based confidence interval.

A confidence interval can also be calculated in the usual way by using an estimate of the variance of the MH-estimate (Greenland & Robins 1985). For this kind of data, the variance is calculated as:

$$var(\ln R\hat{R}_{MH}) \approx \frac{\sum A_i R_{1i} R_{0i}/R_i^2}{[\sum A_{1i} R_{0i}/R_i][\sum A_{0i} R_{1i}/R_i]}$$

The confidence interval is calculated, as before:

$$RR_{MH,L,U} = \exp[\ln R\hat{R}_{MH} \pm 1.96\sqrt{var(\ln R\hat{R}_{MH})}\ ]$$

There are various specific algorithms which can be used to determine the maximum-likelihood estimate for this kind of data (Breslow & Day 1988). However, ordinary multivariate methods can also be used. See Chapter 12.

EXAMPLE:

Let us consider a population distributed over two strata:

Stratum 1	Exposure		
	Yes	No	Total
Number of cases	30	5	35
Number of person years	3,000	1,000	4,000

$$R\hat{D}_1 = 5000 \times 10^{-3} \quad var(R\hat{D}_1) \approx 8.333 \times 10^{-6}$$

$$R\hat{R}_1 = 2.000 \quad var(\ln R\hat{R}_1) \approx 0.2333$$

Stratum 2	Exposure		
	Yes	No	Total
Number of cases	30	225	255
Number of person years	1,000	9,000	10,000

$$\hat{RD}_2 = 5000 \times 10^{-3} \quad var(\hat{RD}_2) \approx 3.278 \times 10^{-5}$$

$$\hat{RR}_2 = 1.200 \quad var(\ln \hat{RR}_2) \approx 0.0378$$

By using the methods presented in this section the following analyses can be carried out:

Direct pooling gives:

$$\hat{RD}_{pool} = \frac{\dfrac{1}{8.333 \times 10^{-6}} \, 5.000 \times 10^{-3} + \dfrac{1}{3.278 \times 10^{-5}} \, 5.000 \times 10^{-3}}{\dfrac{1}{8.333 \times 10^{-6}} + \dfrac{1}{3.278 \times 10^{-5}}} =$$

$$= 5.000 \times 10^{-3}$$

$$var(\hat{RD}_{pool}) \approx \frac{1}{\dfrac{1}{8.333 \times 10^{-6}} + \dfrac{1}{3.278 \times 10^{-5}}} = 6.644 \times 10^{-6}$$

$$RD_{pool,L,U} = 5.000 \times 10^{-3} \pm 1.96 \sqrt{6.644 \times 10^{-6}} =$$

$$= -5.21 \times 10^{-5}, \ 1.01 \times 10^{-2}$$

$$\hat{RR}_{pool} = \exp\left[\dfrac{\dfrac{1}{0.233} \times \ln 2.000 + \dfrac{1}{0.03778} \times \ln 1.200}{\dfrac{1}{0.2333} + \dfrac{1}{0.03778}}\right] =$$

$$= e^{\,0.2535} = 1.289$$

$$var(\ln\hat{RR}_{pool}) \approx \dfrac{1}{\dfrac{1}{0.2333} + \dfrac{1}{0.03778}} = 0.03251$$

$$RR_{pool,L,U} = \exp[\ln 1.289 \pm 1.96 \sqrt{0.03251}\,] =$$

$$= e^{\,-0.09951,\ 0.6073} = 0.905, \ 1.84$$

The Mantel-Haenszel method gives:

$$\hat{RR}_{MH} = \dfrac{30 \times 1000/4000 + 30 \times 9000/10000}{5 \times 3000/4000 + 225 \times 1000/10000} = 1.314$$

$$var(\ln \hat{RR}_{MH}) \approx$$

$$\approx \frac{35 \times 3000 \times 1000/4000^2 \ + \ 255 \times 1000 \times 9000/10000^2}{(30 \times 1000/4000 \ + \ 30 \times 9000/10000)(5 \times 3000/4000 \ + \ 225 \times 1000/10000)} =$$

$$= 0.03259$$

$$RR_{MH,L,U} = \exp[\ln 1.314 \pm 1.96 \sqrt{0.03259}\,] =$$

$$e^{-0.08074, \ 0.6269} = 0.922, \ 1.87$$

$$z = \frac{(30 + 30) \ - \ (35 \times 3000/4000 \ + \ 255 \times 1000/10000)}{\sqrt{35 \times 3000/4000 \times 1000/4000 \ + \ 255 \times 1000/10000 \times 9000/10000}} =$$

$$= 1.519$$

The test-based confidence interval is:

$$RR_{MH,L,U} = 1.314^{1 \pm 1.96/1.519} = 0.924, \ 1.87$$

The maximum likelihood method would give:

$$\hat{RR}_{ML} = 1.298; \quad var(\ln\hat{RR}_{ML}) = 0.02959$$

$$RR_{ML,L,U} = 0.927, \ 1.82$$

7.2.3 Cumulative Incidence

We will now go through the same methods as in the previous section, but this time adapted for studies based on cumulative incidence. The notations used for the stratified analysis of cumulative incidence are the same as for the analysis of cumulative incidence with non-stratified material (see Chapter 6), however, again, with the addition of a subscript i which specifies the stratum in question. For stratum i the following symbols are used:

| | Exposure | | |
	Yes	No	Total
Diseased	A_{1i}	A_{0i}	A_i
Not diseased	$N_{1i} - A_{1i}$	$N_{0i} - A_{0i}$	$N_i - A_i$
Total	N_{1i}	N_{0i}	N_i

Let us again start with pooling. In stratum i the effect is estimated:

$$\hat{RD}_i = \hat{CI}_{1i} - \hat{CI}_{0i}$$

when it is defined as the difference between two cumulative incidences. Its variance is estimated:

$$var(\hat{RD}_i) \approx \frac{\hat{CI}_{1i}(1 - \hat{CI}_{1i})}{N_{1i}} + \frac{\hat{CI}_{0i}(1 - \hat{CI}_{0i})}{N_{0i}}$$

all in accordance with the results in the previous chapter (see Section 6.2.1).

The pooled estimator of the difference is thus:

$$\hat{RD}_{pool} = \frac{\sum \dfrac{1}{\dfrac{\hat{CI}_{1i}(1 - \hat{CI}_{1i})}{N_{1i}} + \dfrac{\hat{CI}_{0i}(1 - \hat{CI}_{0i})}{N_{0i}}} \times \hat{RD}_i}{\sum \dfrac{1}{\dfrac{\hat{CI}_{1i}(1 - \hat{CI}_{1i})}{N_{1i}} + \dfrac{\hat{CI}_{0i}(1 - \hat{CI}_{0i})}{N_{0i}}}}$$

and the variance is:

$$var(\hat{RD}_{pool}) \approx \frac{1}{\sum \dfrac{1}{\dfrac{\hat{CI}_{1i}(1 - \hat{CI}_{1i})}{N_{1i}} + \dfrac{\hat{CI}_{0i}(1 - \hat{CI}_{0i})}{N_{0i}}}}$$

An approximate 95% confidence interval is calculated as:

$$RD_{pool,L,U} = \hat{RD}_{pool} \pm 1.96\sqrt{var(\hat{RD}_{pool})}$$

The principles for analyzing the relative risk for cumulative incidences are also the same as before. Again, the results in the previous chapter form the basis for the stratum-specific expressions (see Section 6.2.2). The relative risk in stratum i is estimated:

$$\hat{RR}_i = \frac{\hat{CI}_{1i}}{\hat{CI}_{0i}}$$

and the variance for the logarithm of this estimator is calculated:

$$var(\ln \hat{RR}_i) \approx \frac{N_{1i} - A_{1i}}{N_{1i}} \frac{1}{A_{1i}} + \frac{N_{0i} - A_{0i}}{N_{0i}} \frac{1}{A_{0i}}$$

The pooled estimator is consequently:

$$\hat{RR}_{pool} = e^{\ln \hat{RR}_{pool}} =$$

$$\exp \left[\frac{\sum \frac{1}{\dfrac{N_{1i} - A_{1i}}{N_{1i}} \dfrac{1}{A_{1i}} + \dfrac{N_{0i} - A_{0i}}{N_{0i}} \dfrac{1}{A_{0i}}} \ln \hat{RR}_i}{\sum \frac{1}{\dfrac{N_{1i} - A_{1i}}{N_{1i}} \dfrac{1}{A_{1i}} + \dfrac{N_{0i} - A_{0i}}{N_{0i}} \dfrac{1}{A_{0i}}}} \right]$$

and its variance is:

$$var(\ln \hat{RR}_{pool}) \approx \frac{1}{\sum \dfrac{1}{\dfrac{N_{1i} - A_{1i}}{N_{1i}} \dfrac{1}{A_{1i}} + \dfrac{N_{0i} - A_{0i}}{N_{0i}} \dfrac{1}{A_{0i}}}}$$

By means of estimate and variance the confidence interval is calculated as follows:

$$RR_{pool,L,U} = \exp[\ln \hat{RR}_{pool} \pm 1.96\sqrt{var(\ln \hat{RR}_{pool})}]$$

The Mantel-Haenszel method is used in the same way as for incidence rates, except that the number of person years is replaced by the number of persons (Tarone 1981):

$$\hat{RR}_{MH} = \frac{\sum A_{1i} N_{0i}/N_i}{\sum A_{0i} N_{1i}/N_i}$$

An approximate confidence interval can be calculated by the test-based method, in which case the test variable is obtained by using the Mantel-Haenszel test. The test, but not the estimator, is the same as for case control studies. This gives:

$$z = \frac{A_1 - E(A_1)}{\sqrt{var(A_1)}}$$

where

$$A_1 = \sum_i A_{1i}, \ E(A_1) = \sum_i A_i N_{1i}/N_i$$

and

$$var(A_1) = \sum_i \frac{A_i(N_i - A_i)N_{1i}N_{0i}}{N_i^2(N_i - 1)}$$

With the aid of the z-value from the Mantel-Haenszel test the test-based confidence interval is determined as follows:

$$RR_{MH,L,U} = \hat{RR}_{MH}^{1 \pm 1.96/z}$$

A confidence interval can also be calculated by using an estimate of the variance of the logarithm of the Mantel-Haenszel estimate. For cumulative incidences this variance is (Greenland and Robins 1985):

$$var(\ln\hat{RR}_{MH}) \approx \frac{\sum (A_i N_{1i} N_{0i} - A_{1i} A_{0i} N_i)/N_i^2}{[\sum A_{1i} N_{0i}/N_i][\sum A_{0i} N_{1i}/N_i]}$$

By using this variance, the confidence interval is calculated as:

$$RR_{MH,L,U} = \exp[\ln\hat{RR}_{MH} \pm 1.96 \sqrt{var(\ln\hat{RR}_{MH})}\ ]$$

To calculate the maximum-likelihood estimate, one can, again, either use an algorithm especially devised for this particular purpose or one of the standard programs used for multivariate analyses, chiefly logistic regression (see Chapter 12).

EXAMPLE:

The tables below describe a population divided into two strata.

Stratum 1	Exposure		
	Yes	No	Total
Diseased	30	5	35
Not diseased	2,970	995	3,965
Total	3,000	1,000	4,000

$$\hat{RD}_1 = 5.000 \times 10^{-3} \quad var(\hat{RD}_1) \approx 8.275 \times 10^{-6}$$

$$\hat{RR}_1 = 2.000 \quad var(\ln\hat{RR}_1) \approx 0.2320$$

Stratum 2	Exposure		
	Yes	No	Total
Diseased	30	225	255
Not diseased	970	8,775	9,745
Total	1,000	9,000	10,000

$$\hat{RD}_2 = 5.000 \times 10^{-3} \quad var(\hat{RD}_2) \approx 3.181 \times 10^{-5}$$

$$\hat{RR}_2 = 1.200 \quad var(\ln\hat{RR}_2) \approx 0.03667$$

With the help of the methods introduced in this section the following analyses can be performed:

Pooling gives:

$$\hat{RD}_{pool} =$$

$$= \frac{\dfrac{1}{8.275\times10^{-6}}\times5.000\times10^{-3} + \dfrac{1}{3.181\times10^{-5}}\times5.000\times10^{-3}}{\dfrac{1}{8.275\times10^{-6}} + \dfrac{1}{3.181\times10^{-5}}} =$$

$$= 5.000\times10^{-3}$$

$$var(\hat{RD}_{pool}) \approx \frac{1}{\dfrac{1}{8.275\times10^{-6}} + \dfrac{1}{3.181\times10^{-5}}} = 6.567\times10^{-6}$$

$$RD_{pool, L, U} = 5.000{\times}10^{-3} \pm 1.96\sqrt{6.567{\times}10^{-6}} =$$

$$= -2.26{\times}10^{-5}, \ 0.0100$$

$$\hat{RR}_{pool} = \exp\left[\frac{\dfrac{1}{0.2320}{\times}\ln 2.0000 + \dfrac{1}{0.03667}{\times}\ln 1.200}{\dfrac{1}{0.2320} + \dfrac{1}{0.03667}}\right] =$$

$$= e^{0.2520} = 1.287$$

$$var(\ln\hat{RR}_{pool}) \approx \frac{1}{\dfrac{1}{0.2320} + \dfrac{1}{0.03667}} = 0.03167$$

$$RR_{pool, L, U} = \exp[\ln 1.287 \pm 1.96\sqrt{0.03167}] =$$

$$= e^{-0.09646, \ 0.6011} = 0.908, \ 1.82$$

The Mantel-Haenszel analysis gives:

$$\hat{RR}_{MH} = \frac{30{\times}1000/4000 + 30{\times}9000/10000}{5{\times}3000/4000 + 225{\times}1000/10000} = 1.314$$

$$var(\ln\hat{RR}_{MH}) \approx$$

$$\approx \frac{\begin{array}{l}(35{\times}3000{\times}1000) - 30{\times}5{\times}4000)/4000^2 + \\ (255{\times}1000{\times}9000 - 30{\times}225{\times}10000)/10000^2\end{array}}{(30{\times}1000/4000 + 30{\times}9000/10000){\times}(5{\times}3000/4000 + 225{\times}1000/10000)} =$$

$$= 0.03168$$

$$RR_{MH,L,U} = \exp[\ln 1.314 \pm 1.96\sqrt{0.03168}] =$$

$$= e^{-0.07577,\ 0.6219} = 0.927,\ 1.86$$

$$z = \frac{(30 + 30) - (35 \times 3000/4000 + 255 \times 1000/10000)}{\sqrt{\dfrac{3000 \times 1000 \times 35 \times 3965}{4000^2(4000 - 1)} + \dfrac{1000 \times 9000 \times 225 \times 9745}{10000^2(10000 - 1)}}} = 1.535$$

with the test-based confidence interval:

$$RR_{MH,L,U} = 1.314^{1 \pm 1.96/1.535} = 0.927,\ 1.86$$

The maximum likelihood results are:

$$\hat{RR}_{ML} = 1.307, \quad var(\ln\hat{RR}_{ML}) \approx 0.03045$$

$$RR_{ML,L,U} = 0.928,\ 1.84$$

7.2.4 Prevalence

As has been pointed out earlier, the incidence rate on the one hand and the cumulative incidence and the prevalence on the other, differ in that different fundamental statistical models are used. By using the same model for both the cumulative incidence and the prevalence the analyses will be wholly analogous.

In the previous chapter it was, however, pointed out that if the purpose is to estimate the relative risk defined as the ratio between incidence rates, and if the prevalences are used wholly for logistical reasons, a better estimate is obtained if the prevalence-odds ratio is used. This improvement is of little importance except with very high prevalences. If the prevalence-odds ratio is to be used, then the prevalences should not be analyzed like the cumulative incidences, but rather like odds ratios, in accordance with the principles set out in the following section.

7.2.5 Odds Ratio

The odds ratio is used to estimate the relative risk for data from case-control studies. The same methods are sometimes used in certain cases when analyzing prevalence data. The symbols used are the same as those in the previous chapters, again with the addition of the subscript i to indicate the stratum in question:

	Exposure		
	Yes	No	Total
Cases	a_i	b_i	N_{1i}
Controls	c_i	d_i	N_{0i}
Total	M_{1i}	M_{0i}	T_i

Let us again begin with pooling. The stratum-specific estimate is (see Section 6.4.1):

$$\hat{OR}_i = \frac{a_i\, d_i}{b_i\, c_i}$$

The analyses are performed by logarithm transformation and the variance for the logarithm of the stratum-specific estimate can be estimated (see Section 6.4.2) as follows:

$$var(\ln\hat{OR}_i) \approx \frac{1}{a_i} + \frac{1}{b_i} + \frac{1}{c_i} + \frac{1}{d_i}$$

A pooled estimate is obtained, exactly as before, by weighing with the inverted variances:

$$\hat{OR}_{pool} = e^{\ln\hat{OR}_{pool}} =$$

$$= \exp\left[\frac{\sum \dfrac{1}{\dfrac{1}{a_i} + \dfrac{1}{b_i} + \dfrac{1}{c_i} + \dfrac{1}{d_i}} \ln\hat{OR}_i}{\sum \dfrac{1}{\dfrac{1}{a_i} + \dfrac{1}{b_i} + \dfrac{1}{c_i} + \dfrac{1}{d_i}}}\right]$$

The variance estimate will be:

$$var(\ln\hat{OR}_{pool}) \approx \frac{1}{\sum \dfrac{1}{\dfrac{1}{a_i} + \dfrac{1}{b_i} + \dfrac{1}{c_i} + \dfrac{1}{d_i}}}$$

An approximate 95% confidence interval is calculated as follows:

$$OR_{pool,L,U} = e^{\ln OR_{pool} \pm 1.96 \sqrt{var(\ln OR_{pool})}}$$

As we saw in the introductory section (7.2.1), the Mantel-Haenszel estimate of an odds ratio is obtained as:

$$\hat{OR}_{MH} = \frac{\sum a_i d_i / T_i}{\sum b_i c_i / T_i}$$

and a test variable, which can be used to determine a test-based confidence interval, is obtained as:

$$z = \frac{\sum a_i - \sum M_{1i} N_{1i} / T_i}{\sqrt{\sum \dfrac{N_{1i} N_{0i} M_{1i} M_{0i}}{T_i^2 (T_i - 1)}}}$$

With these results, a 95% test-based confidence interval is obtained as follows:

$$OR_{MH,L,U} = \hat{OR}_{MH}^{\,1 \pm 1.96/z}$$

There is also a version of the variance estimate for the Mantel-Haenszel estimator for odds ratios. This is (Robins et al. 1986):

$$var(\ln\hat{OR}_{MH}) \approx \frac{\Sigma P_i R_i}{2(\Sigma R_i)^2} + \frac{\Sigma(P_i S_i + Q_i R_i)}{2\Sigma R_i \Sigma S_i} + \frac{\Sigma Q_i S_i}{2(\Sigma S_i)^2}$$

where

$$P_i = \frac{a_i + d_i}{T_i} \quad Q_i = \frac{b_i + c_i}{T_i} \quad R_i = \frac{a_i d_i}{T_i} \quad \text{and } S_i = \frac{b_i c_i}{T_i}$$

Again, a 95% confidence interval can be determined by means of the logarithm transformation:

$$OR_{MH,L,U} = \exp[\ln\hat{OR}_{MH} \pm 1.96\sqrt{var(\ln\hat{OR}_{MH})}\,]$$

A maximum-likelihood estimate of the common effect when using odds ratios can, just as for other sorts of data, be obtained either by means of a special algorithm or by using a multivariate model. The main multivariate model used here is the logistic regression.

EXAMPLE:

The tables below show the material from a case control-study. The data is divided into two strata:

Stratum 1	Exposure		
	Yes	No	Total
Cases	30	5	35
Controls	30	10	40
Total	60	15	75

$$\hat{OR}_1 = 2.000 \quad var(\ln \hat{OR}_1) \approx 0.3667$$

Stratum 2	Exposure		
	Yes	No	Total
Cases	30	225	255
Controls	10	90	100
Total	40	315	355

$$\hat{OR}_2 = 1.200 \quad var(\ln \hat{OR}_2) \approx 0.1489$$

Pooling gives:

$$\hat{OR}_{pool} = \exp\left[\frac{\dfrac{1}{0.3667} \ln 2.000 + \dfrac{1}{0.1489} \ln 1.200}{\dfrac{1}{0.3667} + \dfrac{1}{0.1489}} \right] =$$

$$= e^{0.3298} = 1.391$$

$$var(\ln\hat{OR}_{pool}) \approx \cfrac{1}{\cfrac{1}{0.3667} + \cfrac{1}{0.1489}} = 0.1059$$

$$OR_{pool,L,U} = \exp[\ln 1.391 \pm 1.96\sqrt{0.1059}] =$$

$$= \exp^{-0.3078, \ 0.9678} = 0.735, \ 2.63$$

The Mantel-Haenszel method gives:

$$\hat{OR}_{MH} = \frac{30 \times 10/75 + 30 \times 90/355}{5 \times 30/75 + 225 \times 10/355} = 1.392$$

$$var(\ln\hat{OR}_{MH}) \approx$$

$$\approx \frac{(30+10)/75 \times 30 \times 10/75 + (30+90)/355 \times 30 \times 90/355}{2(30 \times 10/75 + 30 \times 90/355)^2} +$$

$$+ \frac{\begin{array}{c}(30+10)/75 \times 5 \times 30/75 + (5+30)/75 \times 30 \times 10/75 + \\ (30+90)/355 \times 225 \times 10/355 + (225+10)/355 \times 30 \times 90/255\end{array}}{2(30 \times 10/75 + 30 \times 90/355)(5 \times 30/75 + 225 \times 10/355)} +$$

$$+ \frac{(5+30/75 \times 5 \times 30/75 + 225 + 225 \times 10/355)^2}{2(5 \times 30/75 + 225 \times 10/355)^2} = 0.1066$$

$$OR_{MH,L,U} = \exp[\ln 1.392 \pm 1.96\sqrt{0.1066}] =$$

$$= e^{-0.3092, \; 0.9707} = 0.734, \; 2.64$$

$$z = \frac{(30+30) - (35\times60/75+255\times40/355)}{\sqrt{\dfrac{60\times15\times35\times40}{75^2(75-1)} + \dfrac{40\times315\times255\times100}{355^2(355-1)}}} = 1.022$$

Thus, the test-based confidence interval is:

$$OR_{MH,L,U} = 1.392^{1 \pm 1.96/1.022} = 0.738, \; 2.63$$

The maximum-likelihood method gives:

$$\hat{OR}_{ML} = 1.401 \quad var(\ln \hat{OR}_{ML}) \approx 1.087$$

$$OR_{ML,L,U} = 0.734, \; 2.67$$

NOTE: In case-control studies, the control group is sometimes matched. Accordingly, for every case one or sometimes several controls are chosen which, in certain specific ways, resemble the case. To avoid systematic errors in the estimation of the relative risk, matched case-control studies must be analyzed with cases and their corresponding controls together. The analysis is conditioned on the outcome for each set of cases and corresponding control or controls (Miettinen 1985; Rothman 1986). One way of carrying out the analysis is to regard the material as stratified by defining each case and corresponding control as a stratum and using the Mantel-Haenszel method. Let us look at a situation where there is one control per case. Here, each stratum consists of exactly one case and one control and there are only four possible outcomes. See the table below. The table also shows, for each of the possible outcomes, the contribution to the numerator and denominator of the Mantel-Haenszel estimator:

	Exposure							
	Yes	No	Yes	No	Yes	No	Yes	No
Cases	1	0	1	0	0	1	0	1
Controls	1	0	0	1	1	0	0	1
ad/T	0		1/2		0		0	
bc/T	0		0		1/2		0	
Number of tables	r		s		t		u	

The Mantel-Haenszel estimator is thus:

$$\hat{OR}_{MH} = \frac{\Sigma a_i d_i / T_i}{\Sigma b_i c_i / T_i} =$$

$$= \frac{r \times 0 + s \times 1/2 + t \times 0 + u \times 0}{r \times 0 + s \times 0 + t \times 1/2 + u \times 0} = \frac{s}{t}$$

It can, similarly, be demonstrated that for the Mantel-Haenszel test:

$$z = \frac{s - t}{\sqrt{s + t}}$$

(In this special case, the Mantel-Haenszel test coincides with a test called the McNemars test (Armitage 1971)).

It is a good idea to compile the material in the following kind of table:

		Control exposed	
		Yes	No
Case	Yes	r	s
exposed	No	t	u

Using the Mantel-Haenszel estimate and test, a test-based confidence interval can be calculated. Multivariate methods can also be used (See Section 8.4).

7.3 STANDARDIZATION

7.3.1 Direct Standardization

The principles for standardization are the same regardless of the measure of disease occurrence used. Let us assume for the moment that we use the incidence rate. A standardized incidence rate is obtained as a weighted mean value of the stratum-specific incidence rates:

$$SI = \Sigma v_i I_i \quad \text{where} \quad \Sigma v_i = 1$$

The weights, v_i, can in principle be chosen arbitrarily, but they must relate to each other so that the sum of the weights is 1. *Standardization* means that the incidence rate is recalculated to what it would have been if the population were distributed across strata in proportion to the distribution in a *standard population,* rather than according to the real distribution; the weights are proportional to the distribution of the standard population. The purpose of this is to obtain two, or sometimes more, incidence rates which are comparable in the sense that the underlying populations are all distributed in the same way across categories of the stratification variable. In this way one controls for confounding from the stratification variable. Standardization is often carried out for basal demographic variables, but the method can of course be used for any variable.

Let index 1 denote an exposed population and 0 an unexposed population. The standardized relative risk is defined as:

$$SRR = \frac{\Sigma v_i I_{1i}}{\Sigma v_i I_{0i}}$$

$$SRR = \sum_i w_i RR_i \quad \text{and} \quad w_i = \frac{v_i I_{0i}}{\sum_j v_j I_{0j}}$$

The SRR can be written as a weighted mean of the stratum-specific RRs similar to how the estimates were written in the previous section. The weights used will, however, be different and will be determined according to quite different principles.

In the previous section, the weights were chosen so that the pooled estimate had as high a precision as possible. The weights here are determined by the distribution in a standard population and the aim is not to obtain a pooled estimate with as high a precision as possible. The aim is rather to estimate the relative risk, assuming that both the exposed and the unexposed are distributed across the stratification variable in the same way as the standard population. The standardization can consequently also be used in situations where there is effect modification, that is, where the measure of effect is assumed to vary across the strata.

A confidence interval for SRR is calculated by use of the logarithm transformation according to the same principle as given earlier, on the condition that the material is sufficiently large. The variance is:

$$var(\ln S\hat{R}R) = var(\ln\Sigma v_i \hat{I}_{1i}) + var(\ln\Sigma v_i \hat{I}_{0i})$$

under the usual conditions (see Chapter 2). By using the formula for the variance for logarithm transformations, (see Section 2.2.3), each of the variances on the right can be written:

$$var(\ln\Sigma_i v_i \hat{I}_i) \approx \frac{\Sigma v_i^2 var(\hat{I}_i)}{(\Sigma v_i \hat{I}_i)^2}$$

Since the variance for the incidence rate is calculated as A/R^2 (see Chapter 5), the variance will be:

$$var(\ln S\hat{R}R) \approx \frac{\Sigma v_i^2 A_{1i}/R_{1i}^2}{[\Sigma_i v_i \hat{I}_{1i}]^2} + \frac{\Sigma v_i^2 A_{0i}/R_{0i}^2}{[\Sigma_i v_i \hat{I}_{0i}]^2}$$

A 95% confidence interval for SRR is calculated as:

$$SRR_{L,U} = \exp[\ln S\hat{R}R \pm 1.96\sqrt{var(\ln S\hat{R}R)}\ ]$$

The only difference when cumulative incidence or prevalence is used instead of the incidence rate, is that the variance will be different. Using the same symbols as before, and when the relative risk is based on the cumulative incidence, the variance will be:

$$var(\ln S\hat{R}R) \approx \frac{\Sigma v_i^2 \dfrac{A_{1i}}{N_{1i}}\left(1 - \dfrac{A_{1i}}{N_{1i}}\right)/N_{1i}}{[\Sigma_i v_i \hat{CI}_{1i}]^2} +$$

$$+ \frac{\Sigma v_i^2 \dfrac{A_{0i}}{N_{0i}}\left(1 - \dfrac{A_{0i}}{N_{0i}}\right)/N_{0i}}{[\Sigma_i v_i \hat{CI}_{0i}]^2}$$

The confidence interval is calculated by means of this variance estimate in exactly the same way as for incidence rate data. When prevalence is used, the procedure is identical to that used for the cumulative incidence.

EXAMPLE:

Consider a population distributed across two strata:

Stratum 1	Exposure		
	Yes	No	Total
Number of cases	30	5	35
Number of person years	3,000	1,000	4,000

$$\hat{I}_{11} = \frac{30}{3000} = 0.01000 \qquad \hat{I}_{01} = \frac{5}{1000} = 0.005000$$

Stratum 2	Exposure		
	Yes	No	Total
Number of cases	30	225	255
Number of person years	1,000	9,000	10,000

$$\hat{I}_{12} = \frac{30}{1000} = 0.03000 \qquad \hat{I}_{02} = \frac{225}{9000} = 0.02500$$

If the exposed population is taken as the standard population, the standardized relative risk is estimated as:

$$S\hat{R}R = \frac{\frac{3}{4}\times0.01000 + \frac{1}{4}\times0.03000}{\frac{3}{4}\times0.00500 + \frac{1}{4}\times0.02500} = 1.500$$

and the variance as:

$$var(\ln S\hat{R}R) \approx \frac{\left(\dfrac{3}{4}\right)^2 \times \dfrac{30}{3000^2} + \left(\dfrac{1}{4}\right)^2 \times \dfrac{30}{1000^2}}{0.01500^2} +$$

$$+ \frac{\left(\dfrac{3}{4}\right)^2 \times \dfrac{5}{1000^2} + \left(\dfrac{1}{4}\right)^2 \times \dfrac{225}{9000^2}}{0.01000^2} = 0.04653$$

An approximate 95% confidence interval is calculated as:

$$SRR_{L,U} = \exp[\ln 1.500 + 1.96\sqrt{0.04653}] = 0.982, 2.29$$

7.3.2 Indirect Standardization

In certain situations, one of the two populations to be compared cannot be standardized as above. This is usually because the exposed group is so small that stratum-specific figures cannot be calculated in a meaningful way. It can, however, still be possible to standardize the unexposed population with the exposed as standard population. In general, this is carried out so that the observed number of cases in the exposed population is compared with an expected number of cases; the latter is calculated from the stratum-specific figures in the unexposed group and the actual distribution across strata in the exposed group. When this method is used, the whole country or a whole county, possibly with some restrictions, is often used as the unexposed group.

To use the conventional symbols, this time let the observed number of exposed cases be denoted by O. As earlier, the time at risk in the $i{:}te$ stratum in the exposed population is denoted by R_{1i}. I_{0i} is the incidence rate in the $I{:}te$ stratum in the unexposed population. The expected number of cases, E, is calculated as:

$$E = \Sigma R_{1i} I_{0i}$$

The standardized measure of effect is written in this situation as SMR (standardized morbidity ratio) and is estimated:

$$SM\hat{R} = \frac{O}{E}$$

When E is calculated from the incidence rate for the whole country or another large population, E can be assumed to be constant. That means that the confidence interval for the SMR is wholly determined by the distribution of O. A confidence interval for SMR is therefore based on a confidence interval for the mean value of O, $E(O)$; the confidence interval for the SMR is obtained by dividing the two limits by the constant, E. That is:

$$SMR_{L,U} = \frac{E(O)_L}{E}, \quad \frac{E(O)_U}{E}$$

With incidence rates, the confidence interval of the mean value of O is based on the Poisson distribution. This can either be obtained exactly or by means of the normal distribution approximation. The principles are the same as when calculating confidence intervals for the incidence rate (see Section 5.1). This method is often used with small materials, in which case the exact method should be used.

EXAMPLE:

Assume that 15 cases have been observed in a population and that the expected number of cases is calculated as 10. This gives:

$$SM\hat{R} = \frac{15}{10} = 1.500$$

A 95% exact confidence interval for the mean of the observed number of cases will be 8.395, 24.74 according to the table in Appendix 1. The confidence interval for SMR will be:

$$SMR_{L,U} = \frac{8.395}{10}, \quad \frac{24.74}{10} = 0.840, \ 2.47$$

The principles for calculating confidence intervals for the *SMR* is the same as above whether the basic data refers to cumulative incidence or prevalence, but the confidence interval around the mean value of the observed number of cases is calculated from the binomial distribution instead of the Poisson distribution. Here too the main principles are the same as when calculating confidence intervals around the corresponding descriptive measures, i.e., the cumulative incidence or the prevalence (see Sections 5.2 and 5.3).

Chapter 8

MULTIVARIATE MODELS

"Black holes ain't so black."

Hawking SW: A Brief History of Time. From the Big Bang to Black Holes. Bantam Books 1988.

8.1 AIMS AND GENERAL PRINCIPLES

A *multivariate model* is a mathematical model which describes how a number of variables and their parameters specify a stochastic variable. A simple model, which really does not merit the epithet multivariate, is:

$$I = \alpha + \beta X$$

where I, as before, is the (theoretical) incidence rate and X the level of exposure. The slope coefficient, ß, in the model indicates how the incidence rate is affected by a change of one unit in X: for every increase in X of one unit, the incidence rate increases by ß. This model is said to be *linear* or *additive*. Note that the unit in which the incidence rate is measured determines the magnitude of ß and consequently how a ß-value is to be interpreted.

If the exposure is dichotomous and $X = 0$ for the unexposed and $X = 1$ for the exposed, then α is the incidence rate for the unexposed and β the difference in incidence rate between the exposed and the unexposed:

$$RD = I_1 - I_0 = (\alpha + \beta \times 1) - (\alpha + \beta \times 0) = \beta$$

The relative risk is:

$$RR = \frac{\alpha + \beta \times 1}{\alpha + \beta \times 0} = 1 + \frac{\beta}{\alpha}$$

The corresponding *multiplicative model* is:

$$I = \alpha e^{\beta X}$$

According to this model, I increases by a factor of $exp(\beta)$ when X increases by one unit. A multiplicative model is always additive when it is logarithmized:

$$\ln I = \ln \alpha + \beta X$$

If, again, X is dichotomous, then:

$$RD = \alpha e^{\beta} - \alpha e^{0} = \alpha(e^{\beta} - 1)$$

and

$$RR = \frac{\alpha e^{\beta}}{\alpha e^{0}} = e^{\beta}$$

The β of the multiplicative model thus corresponds to the relative risk defined, as before, by the relation $RR = exp(\beta)$.

It is important that the purpose of a multivariate model is clear before it is constructed, since different purposes can lead to greatly differing models. One purpose can be to construct a model which can be used to predict which individuals are going to develop a disease. Another can be to try to explain as much of the variation in disease occurrence as possible. However, the most common purpose in epidemiology is to allow for confounding and effect modification when analyzing the association between exposure and disease; it is in this context that we will discuss multivariate models. This means, for example, that a multivariate model can be a good model even if it only describes some of the variations in the incidence of disease — which is of course almost always the case, since so little is known about the aetiology of most diseases.

To demonstrate how a multivariate model can be used to allow for confounding, the model above can be developed into:

$$I = \alpha + \beta_1 X_1 + \beta_2 X_2$$

where index 1 and 2 denote two different risk factors. As the model shows, β_1 represents the increase in incidence rate when X_1 increases by one unit, on the condition that X_2 remains unchanged. This is exactly what is meant by the effect of X_1 being studied, controlling for confounding by X_2.

Effect modification means that the magnitude of the effect varies when a third variable varies. In the above model there is no effect modification (as long as the effect is measured on the additive scale, that is by RD), since the effect of a change of X_1 is always the same, irrespective of the value of X_2. On the other hand, effect modification will occur if the model is rewritten as follows:

$$I = \alpha + \beta_1 X_1 + \beta_2 X_2 + \beta_3 X_1 X_2$$

In this model, the effect of a change in X_1 is obtained as the sum of the change in the second and the last terms of the model. The last term is determined not only by X_1, but also X_2.

The reason for using multivariate models has here been explained similarly to that for stratified analysis. This means that models should be constructed according to the same principles as those for specifying a stratified analysis. Decisive for whether a particular variable should be included in the model as a confounder is whether it really is a confounder. This can be evaluated by studying the parameter which describes the effect of the exposure; if it remains unchanged when a variable is added or removed then the variable in question is not a confounder. Multivariate models are less sensitive than stratified data for sparse data. One can therefore err on the side of generosity and when in doubt include a variable in the model.

It is easy to test models with various kinds of effect modification when multivariate models are being constructed. However, the potential for simple interpretations of the parameter which describes the effect is reduced when the model includes effect modification; the effect will then vary depending on the value of the effect modifying variable. Consequently, the principles used here also follow those for stratified analysis: models are generally constructed without effect modification unless there are strong reasons for including it. Such reasons can either be that the observed material clearly indicates that a model without effect modification is inadequate or that one has a particular interest in studying the effect modification. Here, it is important to remember that effect modification in a multivariate model cannot simply be interpreted as interaction or synergism in a biological model (Greenland 1979). See Chapter 9.

In the above models, X occurs as a continuous as well as a dichotomous variable. It is of course excellent if the model which includes continuous variables is actually suitable for your data. However, if this is not the case, X can be categorized so that it becomes dichotomous, in which case the incidence rate changes stepwise at the point where X changes its value. For example, in the first model given above, the use of a continuous X variable means that the incidence rate changes with increased exposure at the same rate for all levels of exposure. This is often too strict an assumption, and variables in epidemiological analyses are therefore often dichotomized.

When one wants more than two levels for a variable, one uses so called *indicator- or dummy variables*. Let us look again at the model:

$$I = \alpha + \beta_1 X_1 + \beta_2 X_2$$

If you want to divide the variable X_2 into three intervals, that is, if you want to divide the material into three strata, letting the incidence rate change stepwise between these, one can define the indicator variables X_3 and X_4 in the following way:

X_2	X_3	X_4
interval 1	0	0
interval 2	1	0
interval 3	0	1

The above model can then be replaced by the following, which does not assume that there is a linear change of I when X_2 is changed:

$$I = \alpha + \beta_1 X_1 + \beta_3 X_3 + \beta_4 X_4$$

In accordance with the model, β_3 is added to the earlier terms for the X_2-values within interval 2 and β_4 is added for values within interval 3. The incidence rate thus changes in steps from one stratum to the next.

The above is a fairly general discussion but it nevertheless serves to illustrate certain principles for the use of multivariate models in epidemiological analyses. When selecting a multivariate model for a specific situation there are a considerable number of alternatives to choose from. In the following three sections, some of these will be discussed in connection with various kinds of epidemiological data.

8.2 INCIDENCE RATES

In earlier chapters we based the statistical analysis of incidence rates on the Poisson distribution. A model which is linked to this and frequently used is the *multiplicative Poisson model*. Since the multiplicative model becomes linear when it is logarithmized, it is also an example of a *log-linear model*. For this kind of model the material must be stratified so that the number of cases and the number of person years can be calculated in various strata. (See, e.g., Breslow and Day 1975; Breslow et al. 1983; Breslow 1984). An example of a model which is based, instead, on continuous variables is the *"proportional hazards"* model (Cox 1972). For a detailed discussion of these models we refer the reader to Breslow and Day (1988).

As before, let I be the theoretical incidence rate and R the number of person years at risk. According to the multiplicative Poisson model, the number of cases follows a Poisson distribution with a parameter which is specified as:

$$IR = \alpha e^{\beta X} \quad \text{or} \quad \ln IR = \ln \alpha + \beta X$$

This model is to all intents and purposes, the same as those which were discussed at the beginning of the previous section. Further variables can be added to the model as confounders or as effect modifiers if necessary. If the exposure, X, is a dichotomous variable, the relative risk is obtained as $exp(\beta)$. Most of the computer programs used to estimate the parameters of the model work with the logarithmized model. This means that the parameters obtained must be exponentiated before one can interpret them in epidemiological terms. The parameters of a model are usually estimated iteratively by using the maximum-likelihood method.

The model can be formulated in such a way that both the exposure and the confounding variables are dichotomous and so that effect modification is not included. The resulting model is identical to the one which is implicitly used for the corresponding stratified analysis when the relative risk is assumed to be constant across strata (see Chapter 7). This means that the computer program used for this multivariate model can also be used to determine maximum-likelihood estimates in the corresponding stratified analysis.

8.3 Cumulative Incidence

One model which has come to be used a great deal in epidemiology is *multivariate logistic regression*. This was developed in connection with the famous cardiovascular epidemiological study in Framingham, USA (see, for example, Walker and Duncan 1967). The model stipulates that a probability p, is:

$$p = \frac{1}{1 + \dfrac{1}{e^{\alpha + \beta_1 X_1 + \beta_2 X_2 + \dots}}}$$

This expression can be transformed to:

$$\ln \frac{p}{1 - p} = \alpha + \beta_1 X_1 + \beta_2 X_2 + \dots$$

The transformation, which is performed when the odds are calculated and logarithmized, is called logit; hence the name logistic regression. In analyses of cumulative incidence, the cumulative incidence is set as $CI = p$.

To illustrate a simple application of this model, let the exposure again be dichotomous, with $X = 1$ for exposed and $X = 0$ for unexposed. If the cumulative incidence for exposed and unexposed is defined as CI_1 and CI_0 respectively, the logarithm for the odds-ratio is written as:

$$\ln\left[\frac{\dfrac{CI_1}{1-CI_1}}{\dfrac{CI_0}{1-CI_0}}\right] = \ln\left[\frac{CI_1}{1-CI_1}\right] - \ln\left[\frac{CI_0}{1-CI_0}\right] =$$

$$= (\alpha + \beta_1 \times 1 + \beta_2 X_2 + ...) - (\alpha + \beta_1 \times 0 + \beta_2 X_2 + ...) = \beta_1$$

As the logarithm for the odds-ratio equals β_1, the odds-ratio equals $exp(\beta_1)$, in other words:

$$\frac{\dfrac{CI_1}{1-CI_1}}{\dfrac{CI_0}{1-CI_0}} = e^{\beta_1}$$

This means that when the cumulative incidence is so low that

$$\frac{\dfrac{CI_1}{1-CI_1}}{\dfrac{CI_0}{1-CI_0}} \approx \frac{CI_1}{CI_0}$$

the relative risk, defined as the ratio between the two cumulative incidences, can be approximated:

$$RR \approx e^{\beta_1}$$

This model can be constructed in many different ways, keeping in mind the discussions in the introductory section of this chapter.

8.4 CASE-CONTROL STUDIES

Multivariate logistical regression has become the leading multivariate model for use with case-control studies. For a detailed discussion of this model, we refer the reader to Breslow and Day 1980. In case-control studies the odds ratio is used to estimate the relative risk. One can therefore use logistic regression in essentially the same way as was shown in the previous section. One difference is that the assumption about low probabilities is not required for case-control studies, since the odds ratio is actually the parameter which corresponds to the ratio between the two incidence rates; the odds ratio is not used here as an approximation of the ratio between two proportions, but as the parameter of interest.

The usual fourfold table is completely symmetrical, so that the exposure odds ratio is the same as the case-control odds ratio:

	Exposure		
	Yes	No	Total
Cases	a	b	N_1
Controls	c	d	N_0
Total	M_1	M_0	T

$$\hat{OR} = \frac{a/d}{c/d} = \frac{a/c}{b/d}$$

We have seen that the odds ratio which can be established from the probability of exposure among cases and controls corresponds to the ratio between incidence rates among exposed and unexposed. As a result of the above symmetry however, the probability which is modelled by the logistic model can instead be taken as the probability that an individual is a case (Breslow and Powers 1978). The parameter in the model which corresponds to the exposure will in this case describe how the relative risk is influenced by a change in exposure.

$$\ln OR = \beta \quad \text{and} \quad OR = e^{\beta}$$

It is, again, important to remember that ß describes the effect of a change in exposure of one unit. If the exposure variable is dichotomous, $exp(\beta)$ can be interpreted in the same way as in Chapters 6 and 7. On the other hand, if the exposure variable is continuous, then the scale determines how a ß-value is to be evaluated.

EXAMPLE:

Let the exposure in question be systolic blood pressure measured in mm Hg and let $exp(\beta) = 1.01$. The relative risk is thus 1.01 if the blood pressure rises by 1 mm Hg.

The programs used to estimate the model's parameters produce iterative maximum-likelihood estimates of the ß-values. These must be exponentiated before they can be interpreted in epidemiological terms. The programs also give the *standard deviation* (the square root of the variance) for each ß-estimate. The confidence intervals for the odds ratios are thus calculated in the same way as for the logarithmized variables in Chapters 6 and 7:

$$OR_{L,U} = e^{\beta \pm 1.96\sqrt{var(\beta)}}$$

EXAMPLE:

Let us look again at the case-control example in Chapter 7. Define Y as 1 for cases and as 0 for controls, define X_1 as 1 for exposed and 0 for others, and define X_2 as 1 for individuals in stratum 1 and as 0 for others. Let N be the number of individuals having a specific combination of these variables. The material can then be presented as:

Y	X_1	X_2	N
1	1	1	30
1	0	1	5
0	1	1	30
0	0	1	10
1	1	0	30
1	0	0	225
0	1	0	10
0	0	0	90

In this example, one can formulate the following logistic model:

$$\ln\left[\frac{P(Y = 1)}{1 - P(Y = 1)}\right] = \alpha + \beta_1 X_1 + \beta_2 X_2$$

α corresponds to the probability of being a case among the unexposed in stratum 2 and is determined by the design of the study; α is therefore of no real interest. β_1 corresponds to the effect of the exposure and, in line with our earlier reasoning, $exp(\beta_1) = OR$. Similarly, β_2 corresponds to the effect of the stratification variable; if the stratification variable is exclusively regarded as a confounder, β_2 is of no interest, but if the stratification variable is another exposure under study, β_2 is interpreted in the same way as β_1. The following estimates are thus obtained:

i	β_i	$\sqrt{var(\beta_i)}$	$\hat{OR}_i$	$OR_{i,L,U}$	
1	0.3369	0.3297	1.401	0.734	2.67
2	-1.305	0.3499	0.2712	0.137	0.539

These results are identical to those which were obtained from the maximum-likelihood estimate in the stratified analysis in the example in Chapter 7. It demonstrates how the logistic model can be specified so that it performs the same analysis as a stratified analysis, and how general programs for multivariate models can be used to calculate maximum-likelihood estimates in stratified material.

In the above example, the material was divided into two strata. One indicator variable is sufficient for this. We saw earlier that two indicator variables were needed to stratify the material into three strata. The number of indicator variables should be one less than the number of strata.

We have mentioned before that matched case-control studies should be analyzed with cases and matching controls together. This also applies to logistic regression (see Breslow and Day 1980). Each set of cases and matching controls is thus regarded as one stratum. However, one cannot use the model given above because the ratio between the number of observations and the number of estimated parameters is too low. The number of parameters to be estimated is the number of strata minus one, to which comes the parameters which correspond to exposure and other possible confounders or effect modifiers. One can, however, use *conditional logistic regression*. By making the regression conditional on the total number of exposed in each stratum, the need to estimate those parameters that are associated with the indicator variables will disappear. This method also makes it possible to take into account any potential confounders which were not included in the matching.

Chapter 9

ANALYSIS OF EFFECT MODIFICATION AND SYNERGISM

"It turns out to be very difficult to devise a theory to describe the universe all in one go."

Hawking SW: A Brief History of Time. From the Big Bang to the Black Holes. Bantam Books 1988.

In Chapter 7 effect modification was defined as the effect of an exposure varying with a third variable. Effect modification by age occurs, for example, if the relative risk increases with rising age. An example in Section 7.1.1 illustrated that a consequence of this definition is that the effect modification depends on how the effect is measured. In the example, an effect modification was present if the effect was measured as the difference in occurrence of disease between exposed and unexposed, but not if the effect was measured as the ratio between the occurrence of disease among exposed and unexposed, that is the relative risk (see the example below). Consequently, the presence or absence of effect modification depends on the criterion chosen. The choice lies mainly between the additive and the multiplicative scale.

The fact that the stratum-specific relative risks are constant means therefore that there is no effect modification when the multiplicative scale is used. When this is the case there is usually, instead, an effect modification if the additive scale had been used. Again, see the example. This must also be kept in mind when one is interpreting the results of multivariate modelling. The multivariate logistic regression model, for example, is an example of a multiplicative model. This can be seen from the fact that it becomes additive when logarithmized. A consequence of this is that a logistic model without interaction term has no effect modification with multiplicativity as criterion but usually with additivity as criterion.

So far our discussion here has been about effect modification and we have not considered whether additivity, multiplicativity or possibly some other functional link is the most suitable basis for evaluation.

The term *synergism* is reserved here for effect modification evaluated in a biologically or medically meaningful way. In the pie chart, synergistic causes can be defined as contributing causes which are included in the same "pie" (Rothman 1976; Rothman 1986; Ahlbom & Norell 1986). It can be shown that this definition leads to deviations away from additivity as the criterion for synergism.

EXAMPLE:

The material in the example from Chapter 7 just mentioned can be summarized in the following table, with incidence rates expressed as number of cases per 1,000 person years:

Exposure	Males	Females
Yes	4.0	2.0
No	2.0	1.0
RR	2.0	2.0
RD	2.0	1.0

The effect of the exposure is uniform when the relative risk is used, but not when the difference is used. Hence, synergism is present between exposure and gender.

Let us use the symbols as in the table below:

	Exposure 2	
Exposure 1	Yes	No
Yes	I_{11}	I_{10}
No	I_{01}	I_{00}

The occurrence of synergism is evaluated by comparing the actual incidence rate for the "doubly exposed" with that which would be expected in the absence of synergism. Without synergism:

$$I_{11} - [I_{10} + (I_{01} - I_{00})] = 0$$

One might imagine that this would lead to problems in case-control studies where the relative risks only, and not the actual incidence rates, can be estimated. However, if each term in the expression above is divided by I_{00} one obtains:

$$RR_{11} - [RR_{10} + (RR_{01} - 1)] = 0$$

The presence of synergism can thus also be evaluated on the basis of relative risks obtained, for example, in a case-control study. The material is then best presented in a table of the type below. Note that the reference category is always the doubly unexposed:

	Exposure 2	
Exposure 1	Yes	No
Yes	RR_{11}	RR_{10}
No	RR_{01}	RR_{00}

Various measures of the degree of synergism, *synergy index*, have been suggested (Rothman 1976; Walker 1981). In analogy with the aetiological fraction, a synergy index can, for example, be calculated as the proportion of those new cases which can be attributed to a concurrence between the causes of the disease in question.

Chapter 10

SEVERAL EXPOSURE LEVELS

"Sigtrygg's blow struck Orm in the side, piercing his chain shirt and causing a deep wound; but Orm's sword buried itself in Sigtrygg's throat, and a great shout filled the hall as the bearded head flew from its shoulders, bounced on the edge of the table and fell with a splash into the butt of ale that stood at its feet."

Bengtsson FG: Röde Orm. P.A. Norstedt & Söners Förlag 1941, 1945.

So far we have looked at situations where there are two exposure levels: the individuals have been divided into exposed and unexposed. However, analyses involving three or more exposure levels are frequently preferable. The question of whether or not increased exposure is associated with increased effect is of great importance when evaluating the results of epidemiological studies. When this is the case one usually says that there is a *dose-response relation*. The presence of a dose-response relation, for example, numbered among Hill's well-known "criteria" for evaluating causality (Hill 1965).

The easiest way of carrying out an analysis which takes several exposure levels into account is to analyze each exposure level separately. This means that the individuals in the highest exposure category are compared with the unexposed, then individuals in the next highest category, and so on for all categories of the exposed. Note that the exposed are not compared with the rest of the material but that the reference category rather remains the same the whole time.

When relative risks are compared across different exposure categories it is naturally important that they should be free from confounding. One can, in principle, control for confounding by means of stratified analysis, as in Chapter 7. However, since the various relative risks are going to be compared with each other, it is important that the weights which are used when pooling across strata are the same for all exposure categories. The methods in Chapter 7 which assume that there is a uniform effect across strata, use weights which take into account the precision in each stratum. One cannot, however, be certain that these weights are the same for different exposure categories. There is consequently a risk that the relative risks obtained would not be comparable if they were calculated in this fashion. One way of ensuring that the weights really are the same for all exposure levels is to standardize, rather than to pool with weights that reflect the stratum-specific precision. In such cases one uses direct standardization. See again, Chapter 7.

It is often satisfactory to analyze each exposure level separately if one has a limited number of levels. There is no fundamental difference between dividing a material into exposed and unexposed and dividing it into two levels of exposed as well as into unexposed. However, problems quickly arise when the number of exposure levels increases, because of the fact that the material becomes sparser and the precision of the relative risk estimates is reduced. To counteract the low precision one uses models which simultaneously use information from all exposure categories and which describe how the relative risk increases with increased exposure.

A well-known such method is the Mantel-Haenszel extension test (Mantel 1963). This is a development of the Mantel-Haenszel test which has retained many of the advantages of the latter. The method was developed for case-control studies and is based on each exposure category being allocated a point which is used as an independent variable. Significance tests are no more desirable in dose-response analyses than in other contexts (see Chapter 4). On the other hand, there are not as many obvious alternatives for dose-response analyses as there are for other kinds of analysis, and they have consequently been discussed less.

The multivariate models described in Chapter 8 can also be used when there are several exposure levels. A logistic regression model, for example, can be formulated as follows:

$$\ln \frac{p}{1-p} = \alpha + \beta X$$

with $X = 0, 1, 2, ...$ depending on the exposure category. Just as before, $\exp(\beta)$ is the relative risk when X increases by one unit. One can extend the model with more variables if one wants to control for confounding or analyze effect modification (as discussed in Chapter 7). One should, however, bear in mind

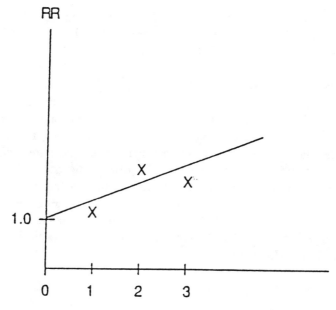

Figure 10.1   A linear regression line is adapted to relative-risk estimates for three levels of exposure.

what was said about standardization earlier in this chapter. According to the above model, the relative risk increases at the same rate across all exposure categories. If this is considered to be too strong an assumption, indicator variables can be used. (See Chapter 7.) In this case, the model can be rewritten as:

$$\ln \frac{p}{1-p} = \alpha + \beta_1 X_1 + \beta_2 X_2 + ...$$

where X_1 and X_2 are indicator variables which identify the respective exposure categories. If, for example, X_1 is defined as 1 for the first exposure category and as 0 otherwise and X_2 as 1 for the second exposure category and as 0 otherwise, then $\exp(\beta_1)$ gives the relative risk for the first exposure category relative to the unexposed group and $\exp(\beta_2)$ similarly gives the relative risk for the second exposure category. This approach solves the problem of not being certain that the increase in risk is uniform across the whole exposure range. In return, the need arises to estimate a parameter for each of the exposure categories above the reference category. To some extent, this approach consequently shares the problem of diminishing precision when the exposure variable is divided into an increasing number of categories. On the other hand this problem is smaller for multivariate models than for the simple stratified analysis.

Rothman (1986) has suggested that a simple linear regression analysis should be used with dose-response analyses. This is then based on separate estimates of the relative risk in the different exposure categories. These can be standardized or controlled for confounding in some other way. The relative risk estimates are the "y-values" of the regression analysis. The corresponding "x-values" are determined by the exposure categories. If the actual exposures in the individual exposure categories are not known, the x-values can be set at 0, 1, ... Since usually the precision of the relative risk estimates for the different exposure categories differ, a weighted regression analysis should be carried out. The weights will be proportional to the inverted variances for the estimates of the relative risks. (See Figure 10.1).

Chapter 11

META ANALYSIS

"Achilles: Don't tell me you believe in fortune-telling! Tortoise: No...but they say it works even if you don't believe in it!"

Hofstadter DR: Gödel, Escher, Bach: An Eternal Golden Braid. Basic Books, Inc. 1979.

It is highly uncommon for a single epidemiological study to allow firm conclusions to be drawn about a link between exposure and illness. Although the situation varies with the amount of a priori information of different origin, several confirmatory studies are typically necessary before a finding can be seen as proven. This is because, generally, neither random nor systematic sources of error can be entirely eliminated when analyzing the results of a study. There is consequently a need for methods which can be used to compare the results of a number of studies, so-called *meta-analysis*. See Greenland (1987) for a survey of such methods.

A major problem with meta-analysis is that the studies which are to be compared with each other vary in design and execution. As a consequence, the comparability of the various studies can be limited. This is partly because they are marred by varying degrees of systematic error, partly because they use different criteria for diagnosis or exposure, for example. No statistical methods for coping with this lack of comparability are available to the epidemiologist. However, the need to pool study results remains, which results in meta-analysis being attempted in spite of the above-mentioned problems. The results of meta-analysis can in such cases not be interpreted mechanically; they must rather be interpreted in conjunction with appraisals of the design and systematic errors of individual studies.

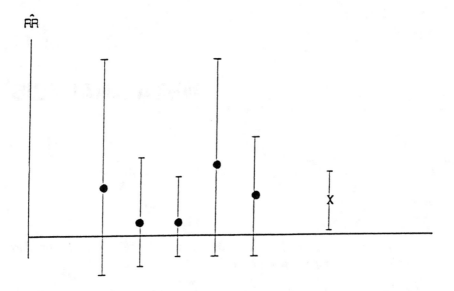

Figure 11.1 The results of five studies of one and the same association are pooled in a meta-analysis.

Chapter 4 contained a lengthy discussion of the problems associated with the use of significance testing for evaluating random error in a study. These problems become particularly obvious in connection with meta-analysis. If one insists on summarizing the results of a study as either significant or non-significant, one might imagine a meta-analysis which tells us how many of the available studies are significant and how many are not significant. Yet this is clearly not an acceptable procedure, as is demonstrated by Figure 11.1, which gives the confidence intervals for five available studies. It is apparent that all the confidence intervals include $RR = 1$. In other words, all five studies are non-significant. At the same time, all five observed relative risks are elevated. It would be absurd merely to establish that five non-significant studies have been carried out and conclude that the data clearly indicates that there is no link between exposure and illness. Nevertheless, this is not an uncommon procedure (Freiman et al. 1978).

A good way of obtaining a basis for comparing the results of various studies is to calculate the confidence intervals for the individual studies and to display them in a figure such as Figure 11.1. There are also methods for carrying out formal comparisons of individual study results, such as by calculating the mean value. It is actually this formal type of comparison which is called meta-analysis.

When calculating the mean of the relative risks from a number of available studies the situation is very similar to the one discussed in Chapter 7, where the results in single strata were pooled to give a summary estimate. One important precondition if this estimate is to be of any use is that the various studies must provide relative risk estimates of one and the same underlying relative risk. If this condition is fulfilled, the methods for stratified analysis given in Chapter 7 are directly applicable. It seems natural to use direct pooling in meta-analysis. Let us assume that there is a series of studies of one and the same association and that:

$$\hat{RR}_i \quad \text{and} \quad var(\ln\hat{RR}_i)$$

is the relative risk estimate and the corresponding variance estimate from the i:th of these. Just as was the case with the stratified analysis, a mean is obtained which takes the precision of the respective relative risk estimates into account as:

$$\hat{RR}_{pool} = \exp\left[\frac{\sum \frac{1}{var(\ln\hat{RR}_i)}\ln\hat{RR}_i}{\sum \frac{1}{var(\ln\hat{RR}_i)}}\right]$$

The variance is taken as:

$$var(\ln\hat{RR}_{pool}) \approx \frac{1}{\sum \frac{1}{var(\ln\hat{RR}_i)}}$$

that is as one over the sum of the weights.

The confidence interval is formed, just as before, by point estimate and variance.

The precondition upon which the calculation of the summary value described here is based, is that every study provides an estimate of one and the same underlying relative risk. Thus, it is not necessary for all the studies to be of the same design. For example, it is no hindrance if some of the pooled studies are cohort studies while others are case-control studies.

The above procedure demands, apart from the information needed to be able to evaluate the validity, a point estimate and a variance for each study. One problem here is that study reports frequently fail to give the variance, and that often only the confidence interval, for example, is available. However, an estimate of the variance can be calculated from the confidence interval. Assuming that a 95% confidence interval for the relative risk is constructed by use of the logarithm transformation, the variance can be estimated as follows:

$$var(\ln R\hat{R}) \approx \left[\frac{\ln RR_U - \ln RR_L}{2 \times 1.96} \right]^2$$

If only a P-value or a test variable is available for a study, a test-based confidence interval can be calculated, after which the required variance can be established approximately, in the way demonstrated above.

Chapter 12

COMPUTER PROGRAMS

"But now we have with us some concepts that greatly alter the whole understanding of things.... It remains to work these concepts into a practical, down-to-earth context, and for this there is nothing more practical or down-to-earth than what I have been talking about along — the repair of an old motorcycle."

Pirsig RM: Zen, and the Art of Motorcycle Maintenance. Vintage 1971.

It is something of an understatement to point out that the 1980s saw enormous developments in the world of computers. At the beginning of the decade, computer computations were generally still being performed on large, main frame, computers, while today powerful personal computers are used for all but the largest materials. Strictly speaking, everyone engaged in epidemiological research ought to have access to a personal computer. This naturally has consequences for the choice of data analysis method. It means, for example, that the easy to use test-based method for determining confidence intervals is of less importance today. At the same time, the iterations which the maximum-likelihood methods demand no longer pose the same problems.

The development of programs has kept pace with that of the computers themselves. Standard programs have been developed for many fields and the programs are now much easier to use. However, analyses for the type of epidemiological data described in this book do not feature among all the general statistical packages yet. Nevertheless, increasing numbers of special programs for epidemiology are becoming available and most epidemiological needs can now be met by what is on the market. Developments in this field are taking place very rapidly and any attempt to describe these runs the risk of being hopelessly out of date by the time it reaches the reader.

As far as we are aware, the first package of programs for epidemiological analyses was devised for use with a Hewlett-Packard desk top calculator (Rothman and Boice 1982). These programs cover many of the epidemiological applications and still played an important role until recently, partly because they are so easy to use. It is, for example, still difficult to find later programs for the exact analyses included in this early package which are anywhere near as easy to use. One problem with the Hewlett-Packard and these exact analyses is of course that the necessary iterations in some cases take a considerable amount of time. The approximate confidence intervals which are calculated are, with certain exceptions, test-based, which with today's potential is perhaps an unnecessarily low level of ambition. Also, of course, data entry poses a problem on any desk top calculator if a full scale study is to be analyzed.

EPILOG is a comprehensive package for personal computers which contains programs for many of the common analyses used in epidemiology. Especially for case control-studies there are some useful programs here, including exact analyses of fourfold tables and unconditional/conditional logistic regression. The program for logistic regression, for example, is easy to use because it automatically creates indicator variables if these are required. One disadvantage with EPILOG in some situations is that a certain amount of experience is necessary before one gets used to the way in which the data is fed in. It cannot, for instance, be entered directly from the keyboard into an analysis program; it must first be stored in a file which is then read by the analysis program.

Certain general-purpose packages can also be used for epidemiological analyses. The popular SAS package, for example, has been supplied with a supplement which can be used for many of the analyses common in epidemiology. GLIM is another general program package which can be made to carry out many of the epidemiological analyses easily and with flexibility. It is, however, advanced and difficult to master.

More recently, programs specifically designed for epidemiological analyses have been introduced. For a review of these we refer the reader to *Epidemiology Monitor* (1987). Several of the programs in this review are so-called "public domain" programs, which means that they may be copied and disseminated. One of these is EPID which is very easy to use and has a wide field of application. It is menu driven with simple instructions, making a manual hardly necessary. Data can be entered straight from the keyboard. Another of these, also easy to use, is LOGRESS, which performs logistic regressions. PDIST is a program which calculates the P-value functions described in Chapter 4 with the aid of normal distribution approximation. MHCHI performs analyses of stratified data from case control studies. The material can be entered from the keyboard. The program calculates Mantel-Haenszel estimates and confidence intervals by the Greenland and Robins' method described in Chapter 7. It further gives a graphic presentation of the entire P-value function.

Appendix 1

Table 1. Exact 95% and 90% confidence intervals for the parameter μ in a Poisson distribution for different observed numbers A.

A	95 % confidence limits		90 % confidence limits	
0	0.000	3.689	0.000	2.996
1	0.025	5.572	0.051	4.744
2	0.242	7.225	0.355	6.296
3	0.619	8.767	0.818	7.754
4	1.090	10.24	1.366	9.154
5	1.623	11.67	1.970	10.51
6	2.202	13.06	2.613	11.84
7	2.814	14.42	3.285	13.15
8	3.454	15.76	3.981	14.44
9	4.115	17.09	4.695	15.71
10	4.795	18.39	5.425	16.96
11	5.491	19.68	6.169	18.21
12	6.201	20.96	6.924	19.44
13	6.922	22.23	7.690	20.67
14	7.654	23.49	8.464	21.89
15	8.395	24.74	9.246	23.10
16	9.145	25.98	10.04	24.30
17	9.903	27.22	10.83	25.50
18	10.67	28.45	11.63	26.69
19	11.44	29.67	12.44	27.88
20	12.22	30.89	13.26	29.06

Table 2. Exact 95% confidence intervals for the parameter p in a binomial distribution for different observed numbers A and different total numbers n.

n	A	1	2	3	4	5
1	.000 .975					
2	.000 .842	.013 .987				
3	.000 .708	.008 .906				
4	.000 .602	.006 .806	.068 .932			
5	.000 .522	.005 .716	.053 .853			
6	.000 .459	.004 .641	.043 .777	.118 .882		
7	.000 .410	.004 .579	.037 .710	.099 .816		
8	.000 .369	.003 .527	.032 .651	.085 .755	.157 .843	
9	.000 .336	.003 .482	.028 .600	.075 .701	.137 .788	
10	.000 .308	.003 .445	.025 .556	.067 .652	.122 .738	.187 .813

APPENDIX 2

EXERCISES

Chapter 2

1. X is a stochastic variable with the probability function

$$p(x) = \begin{cases} 1/4 & \text{for } x=1 \\ 3/4 & \text{for } x=0 \end{cases}$$

Calculate the mean value and the variance.

2. X_1 and X_2 are independent stochastic variables with the same probability functions as above. Give the probability function for

$$Y = X_1 + X_2$$

3. Calculate the mean value and variance for Y in Exercise 2:

a) from the probability function for Y.

b) from the rules for linear combinations.

4. X_1 and X_2 are defined as in Exercise 2. Give the probability function for

$$Y = (X_1 + X_2)/2$$

5. Calculate the mean value and the variance for Y in Exercise 4:

   a) from the probability function for Y.

   b) from the rules for linear combinations.

6. X is a stochastic variable with the frequency function

$$f(x) = \begin{cases} x/2 & \text{for } 0 < x < 2 \\ 0 & \text{otherwise} \end{cases}$$

   a) Draw the frequency function and calculate the area.

   b) Calculate $P(X \leq 1)$ and $P(X > 3/2)$.

7. X is defined as in Exercise 6.

   a) Calculate the mean value and variance.

   b) Give the distribution function of X.

8. $X \sim N(1,4)$. What is

   $P(X > 5)$?

9. X_1 and $X_2 \sim N(0,1)$ and independent. What is

   $P(X_1 + X_2 \leq 2)$?

10. $X \sim bin\ (3, 0.2)$.

   a) Calculate $p(x)$ for $x = 0,...,3$.

   b) What is $\sum\limits_{x=0}^{3} p(x)$?

   c) What is $P(X \geq 2)$?

11. $X \sim bin\ (100, 0.1)$. Calculate $P(X > 90)$.

12. $X \sim$ Poisson (1.5). Calculate $p(x)$ for

   $x = 0, ...$

13. $X \sim$ Poisson (10). Calculate $P(X > 15)$.

14. There are 5 cases and 5 controls. A total of 5 persons have been exposed. X is the number of exposed cases. Calculate $P(X = 1)$ and $P(X \leq 1)$ assuming that X is hypergeometrically distributed.

15. There are 50 cases and 50 controls. A total of 50 persons have been exposed. X is the number of exposed cases. Calculate $P(X \leq 10)$ assuming that X is hypergeometrically distributed.

Chapter 4

16. X is normally distributed with a mean value μ and a variance of 4. A random sample of 16 independent observations gives a mean value of 5.

$$H_0 : \mu = 4 \text{ and } H_1 : \mu > 4$$

a) Calculate the P-value.

b) For which mean value is $P = 0.05$?

17. Take the situation given in Exercise 16, i.e., $X \sim N(\mu,4)$ together with the fact that a random sample of 16 observations gives the mean value 5:

a) Calculate the P-value function and describe it in graphic terms.

b) Which mean values correspond to $P = 0.025$?

18. Of 10 persons, 1 becomes ill. $H_0 : CI$ (the cumulative incidence) $= 0.2$ and $H_1 : CI < 0.2$. Calculate the P-value.

19. Ten out of 100 persons become ill. Of a further 100 persons, 15 become ill. Let CI_1 and CI_2 be the cumulative incidences for the respective groups. $H_0 : CI_1 = CI_2$ and $H_1 : CI_1 < CI_2$.

a) Calculate the P-value from an unconditional analysis.

b) Calculate the P-value by normal distribution approximation based on a conditional analysis.

20. 5 out of 5 persons were exposed. Of a further 5 persons, 4 were exposed. $H_0 : P$ (exposure) is the same in both groups. Calculate an exact P-value from a conditional analysis.

21. $X \sim N(\mu,4)$. An observation of X gives $x_0 = 5$. Construct a 95% confidence interval for μ.

22. X is as above. 4 independent observations of X give a mean value of 5. Construct a 95% confidence interval for μ.

Chapter 5

23. During a certain period of time, A cases occur in a population comprising R person years. Suggest an estimate of the incidence rate. What can be said about the mean value, variance and type of distribution of the estimate?

24. In a study base consisting of 3,000 person years, 20 cases of an illness occurred. Calculate the 95% confidence interval for the incidence rate:

    a) Exactly.

    b) By means of normal distribution approximation.

25. During a particular period of time. A cases occur in a population of N individuals. Suggest an estimate of the cumulative incidence. What can be said about the mean value, variance and type of distribution of the estimate?

26. $X \sim bin(10{,}000, CI)$. One observation of X gives $x_0 = 100$. Construct a 95% confidence interval for CI. Use normal distribution approximation and assume that the variance is stable.

27. In a population consisting of 6,000 individuals, 6 cases of an illness occurred during a particular period of time. Calculate the 95% confidence interval for the cumulative incidence:

a) By normal distribution approximation.

b) By the Poisson approximation.

Chapter 6

28. The table below describes the data from a cohort study

	Exposure		
	Yes	No	Total
Cases	41	15	56
Person years	28,010	19,017	47,027

a) Calculate a 95% confidence interval for RD.

b) Calculate a 95% confidence interval for RR by means of logarithm transformation and normal distribution approximation.

c) Calculate a 95% confidence interval for RR using the test-based method, with the test result obtained from the logarithm transformation in Exercise b.

d) Calculate a 95% confidence interval for *RR* using the test-based method, with the test result obtained from a conditional analysis.

29. The following table was obtained from a cohort study:

	Exposure		
	Yes	No	Total
Cases	30	21	51
Non-cases	174	184	358
Total	204	205	409

a) Calculate a 95% confidence interval for *RD*.

b) Calculate a 95% confidence interval for *RR* by logarithm transformation and normal distribution approximation.

c) Calculate a 95% confidence interval for *RR* using the test-based method and based on a conditional analysis.

30. A case-control study gave the following table:

	Exposure		
	Yes	No	Total
Cases	96	104	200
Controls	109	666	775
Total	205	770	975

a) Calculate a 95% confidence interval for *OR* using Woolf's method.

b) Calculate a 95% confidence interval for *OR* using the test-based method, with the test result obtained from a conditional analysis (with normal distribution approximation of the hypergeometrical distribution).

Chapter 7

31. The table below describes data in a cohort study:

Stratum 1.

	Exposure		
	Yes	No	Total
Cases	32	2	34
Person years	52,407	18,790	71,197

Stratum 2.

	Exposure		
	Yes	No	Total
Cases	104	12	116
Person years	43,248	10,673	53,921

a) Calculate the point estimate of the rate difference and a 95% confidence interval by pooling with weights proportional to the inverted stratum-specific variances.

b) Calculate stratum-specific relative risks and 95% confidence intervals.

c) Calculate the point estimate of the relative risk and a 95% confidence interval by pooling with weights proportional to the inverted variances.

d) Calculate the point estimate of the relative risk in accordance with the Mantel-Haenszel analogy, as well as a 95% test-based confidence interval.

e) Calculate a 95% confidence interval for the relative risk using the estimate in d) with the variance from c).

f) Calculate a 95% confidence interval for the relative risk using the estimate in d) with a variance according to Greenland & Robins.

32. The table below describes the data in a cohort study:

Stratum 1.

	Exposure		
	Yes	No	Total
Cases	8	5	13
Persons	106	120	226

Stratum 2.

	Exposure		
	Yes	No	Total
Cases	22	16	38
Persons	98	85	183

a) Calculate the point estimate of the difference and a 95% confidence interval by pooling with weights proportional to the inverted stratum-specific variances.

b) Calculate stratum-specific relative risks and 95% confidence intervals.

c) Calculate the point estimate of the relative risk and a 95% confidence interval by pooling with weights proportional to the inverted variances.

d) Calculate the point estimate of the relative risk according to the Mantel-Haenszel analogy, as well as a 95% test-based confidence interval.

e) Calculate a 95% confidence interval for the relative risk using the estimate in d) with the variance from c).

f) Calculate a 95% confidence interval for the relative risk using the estimate in d) and with a variance according to Greenland & Robins.

33. A case-control study gave rise to the following data:

Stratum 1.

	Exposure	
	Yes	No
Cases	15	64
Controls	319	1,409

Stratum 2.

	Exposure	
	Yes	No
Cases	8	72
Controls	53	381

a) Calculate stratum-specific odds ratios and 95% confidence intervals.

b) Calculate the point estimate of the odds ratio and a 95% confidence interval by pooling with weights proportional to the inverted variances.

c) Calculate the point estimate of the odds ratio according to the Mantel-Haenszel method and a 95% test-based confidence interval.

34. A case-control study gave the following:

Stratum 1.

	Exposure	
	Yes	No
Cases	10	90
Controls	5	95

Stratum 2.

	Exposure	
	Yes	No
Cases	3	47
Controls	0	50

a) Calculate stratum-specific odds ratios and 95% confidence intervals.

b) Calculate the point estimate of the odds ratio and a 95% confidence interval by pooling with weights proportional to the inverted variances.

c) Calculate the point estimate of the odds ratio according to the Mantel-Haenszel method, as well as a 95% test-based confidence interval.

d) Calculate a 95% confidence interval for the odds ratio using the estimate in c) with a variance according to Robins et al.

35. A matched case-control study gave the following data:

		Control exposed	
		Yes	No
Case exposed	Yes	200	5
	No	1	197

Calculate the point estimate of the odds ratio and a 95% confidence interval.

36. The tables below describe the data from a cohort study:

Stratum 1.

	Exposure		
	Yes	No	Total
Cases	30	5	35
Person years	3,000	1,000	4,000

Stratum 2.

	Exposure		
	Yes	No	Total
Cases	30	225	255
Person years	1,000	9,000	10,000

a) Calculate the standardized relative risk if the unexposed population is chosen as the standard population.

b) Calculate a 95% confidence interval for the standardized relative risk in a).

c) The same data as above is given in an example in Chapter 7.3.1. In that example, we calculated the standardized relative risk with weights from the exposed population. The *SRR* was calculated as 1.50, with the upper and lower limits for the 95% confidence interval being 0.98 and 2.29 respectively. Compare these values with the results from a) and b) above and discuss them.

37. In an *SMR*-analysis of incidence data, $O = 3$ and $E = 1.5$. Calculate the point estimate of the *SMR* and an exact 95% confidence interval.

38. O is Poisson ($SMR \times E$), where $E = 25$. An observation of O gives $O = 30$. Calculate a 95% confidence interval for the *SMR* using normal distribution approximation. Assume that the variance is stable and regard E as a constant.

39. A cohort study gave the following:

	Exposed population			Reference population		
	Person years	Cases	I	Person years	Cases	I
Young	6,000	60	0.010	1,000	5	0.005
Old	2,000	60	0.030	9,000	225	0.025
All	8,000	120	0.015	10,000	230	0.023

a) Calculate the *SMR* and a 95% test-based confidence interval.

b) O is Poisson ($SMR \times E$). Calculate a 95% confidence interval for the SMR. Use normal distribution approximation and assume that the variance is stable and that E can be seen as a constant.

c) O is Poisson ($SMR \times E$). Calculate a 95% confidence interval for the SMR by normal distribution approximation of the logarithm transformation. Regard E as a constant.

d) Calculate a 95% confidence interval based on the assumption that the SMR is a ratio between two standardized incidence rates.

e) Calculate the RR according to the Mantel-Haenszel method and a 95% test-based confidence interval.

f) The confidence intervals calculated in a)–e) differ in size. Discuss possible reasons for this.

40. X is Poisson (μ).

a) Suggest an estimator for μ. What can be said about the mean value and variance of the estimate?

b) Derive the ML-estimate for μ.

41. Derive the ML-estimate for the cumulative incidence.

SOLUTIONS TO THE EXERCISES

1. $p(x) = \begin{cases} 1/4 \text{ for } x = 1 \\ 3/4 \text{ for } x = 0 \end{cases}$

$E(X) = \Sigma \times p(x) = 0 \times 3/4 + 1 \times 1/4 = 1/4$

$var(X) = \Sigma p(x)[x - E(X)]^2 = 3/4 \times (1/4)^2 + 1/4 \times (3/4)^2 =$
$= 1/16(3/4 + 9/4) = 3/16$

2. $Y = X_1 + X_2$

$p(y) = \begin{cases} 1/16 \text{ for } y = 2 \\ 6/16 \text{ for } y = 1 \\ 9/16 \text{ for } y = 0 \end{cases}$

3. a)
$E(Y) = \Sigma y p(y) = 0 \times 9/16 + 1 \times 6/16 + 2 \times 1/16 =$
$= 8/16 = 1/2$

$var(Y) = \Sigma p(y)(y - E(Y))^2 =$
$= 9/16(0-1/2)^2 + 6/16(1-1/2)^2 + 1/16(2-1/2)^2 = 6/16$

b) $E(Y) = E(X_1 + X_2) = E(X_1) + E(X_2) = 2 \times 1/4 = 1/2$

$$var(Y) = var(X_1 + X_2) = var(X_1) + var(X_2) = 6/16$$

4. $Y = 1/2(X_1 + X_2)$

$$p(y) = \begin{cases} 1/16 & \text{for } y = 1 \\ 6/16 & \text{for } y = 1/2 \\ 9/16 & \text{for } y = 0 \end{cases}$$

5. a) $E(Y) = \Sigma y p(y) = 9/16 \times 0 + 6/16 \times 1/2 + 1/16 \times 1 = 1/14$

$$var(Y) = \Sigma p(y)(y - E(Y))^2 =$$
$$= 9/16 \, (0 - 1/4)^2 + 6/16 \, (1/2 - 1/4)^2 + 1/16 \, (1 - 1/4)^2 = 3/32$$

  b)
$$E(Y) = E(1/2 X_1 + 1/2 X_2) = E(1/2 X_1) + E(1/2 X_2) =$$
$$= 1/2 \, E(X_1) + 1/2 \, E(X_2) = 1/4$$

$$var(Y) = var(1/2 X_1 + 1/2 X_2) = 1/4 \, var(X_1) + 1/4 \, var(X_2) =$$
$$= 1/4 \, (2 \times 3/16) = 3/32$$

6. a) $f(x) = \begin{cases} x/2 & \text{for } 0 < x < 2 \\ 0 & \text{otherwise} \end{cases}$

The area under the function $= 1$

b) $P(X \leq 1) = \int_{-\infty}^{1} f(x)dx = \int_{0}^{1} x/2 \ dx = I\!\!\!\Big|_{0}^{1} x^2/4 = 1/4$

$P(X > 3/2) = \int_{3/2}^{\infty} f(x)dx = I\!\!\!\Big|_{3/2}^{2} x^2/4 = 1 - 9/16 = 7/16$

7. a) $E(X) = \int_{-\infty}^{\infty} x \, f(x)dx = \int_{0}^{2} x^2/2 \ dx = I\!\!\!\Big|_{0}^{2} x^3/6 = 4/3$

$var(X) = \int_{-\infty}^{\infty} f(x)(x - E(X))^2 dx = \int_{0}^{2} x/2 \ (x - 4/3)^2 \ dx =$

$= 1/2 \ I\!\!\!\Big|_{0}^{2} x^4/4 - 8x^3/9 + 8x^2/9 = 1/2 \ (4 - 64/9 + 32/9) = 2/9$

b) $F(x) = P(X \leq x) = \int_{-\infty}^{x} f(x)dx$

8. $X \sim N(1,4)$

Transform: $Y = \dfrac{X-1}{\sqrt{4}} \Rightarrow Y \sim N(0,1)$

$P(X > 5) \iff P(Y > 2)$

Table gives $P(Y > 2) = 1 - P(Y \leq 2) = 1 - 0.9773 = 0.0227$

9. $Y = X_1 + X_2 \sim N(0,2)$
    $Z = Y/\sqrt{2} \sim N(0,1)$
    $P(Y \leq 2) = P(Z \leq \sqrt{2}) = 0.921$

10. a) $X \sim bin(3,0.2)$

   i.e. $p(x) = \begin{pmatrix} 3 \\ x \end{pmatrix} \times 0.2^x \times 0.8^{3-x}, \, x = 0, 1, 2, 3$

   $p(0) = \dfrac{3!}{0! \, 3!} \times 0.2^0 \times 0.8^3 = 0.512$

   $p(1) = \dfrac{3!}{1! \, 2!} \times 0.2 \times 0.64 = 0.384$

   $p(2) = \dfrac{3!}{2! \, 1!} \times 0.04 \times 0.8 = 0.0960$

   $p(3) = \dfrac{3!}{3! \, 0!} \times 0.2^3 \times 1 = 0.00800$

   b) The sum is 1.00

   c) $P(X \geq 2) = p(2) + p(3) = 0.104$

11. $X \sim bin\,(100, 0.1)$

$E(X) = 100 \times 0.1 = 10$

$var(X) = 100 \times 0.1 \times 0.9 = 9$

Normal distribution approximation gives:

$X \sim N(10, 9),\ Z = \dfrac{X - 10}{3}$

$P(X > 90) = 1 - P(X \leq 90) = 1 - P(Z \leq 80/3) \approx 0\,(< 10^{-9})$

12. $X \sim \text{Poisson}\,(1.5),\ p(x) = e^{-1.5}\,\dfrac{1.5^x}{x!}$

$p(0) = e^{-1.5} = 0.223$

$p(1) = e^{-1.5} \times 1.5 = 0.335$

$p(2) = e^{-1.5} \times \dfrac{1.5^2}{1 \times 2} = 0.251$

$p(3) = e^{-1.5} \times \dfrac{1.5^3}{1 \times 2 \times 3} = 0.126$

etc.

13. Normal distribution approximation gives:

$$X \sim N(10,10) \rightarrow P(X > 15) \approx P\left(Z > \frac{15-10}{\sqrt{10}}\right) =$$

$$= P(Z > \sqrt{2.5}) = 0.0569$$

Taking into account the fact that the normal distribution is continuous gives:

$$P = P\left(Z > \frac{15.5 - 10}{\sqrt{10}}\right) = 0.0410$$

The exact value is 0.0487

14.
$$p(x) = \frac{\begin{pmatrix} N_1 \\ x \end{pmatrix}\begin{pmatrix} N_0 \\ n-x \end{pmatrix}}{\begin{pmatrix} N \\ n \end{pmatrix}}$$

$$p(1) = \frac{\begin{pmatrix} 5 \\ 1 \end{pmatrix}\begin{pmatrix} 5 \\ 4 \end{pmatrix}}{\begin{pmatrix} 10 \\ 5 \end{pmatrix}} = \frac{\dfrac{5!}{1! \, 4!} \times \dfrac{5!}{4! \, 1!}}{\dfrac{10!}{5! \, 5!}} = \frac{25}{252} = 0.0992$$

$$p(0) = \frac{\begin{pmatrix} 5 \\ 0 \end{pmatrix}\begin{pmatrix} 5 \\ 5 \end{pmatrix}}{\begin{pmatrix} 10 \\ 5 \end{pmatrix}} = \frac{1 \times 1}{252} = 0.00397$$

$$P(X \leq 1) = p(0) + p(1) = 0.103$$

15. X is hyper-geometrically distributed

$$E(X) = n\frac{N_1}{N} = \frac{50 \times 50}{100} = 25$$

$$var(X) = \frac{N_1\,N_0\,n(N-n)}{N^2(N-1)} = \frac{50^4}{100^2 \times 99}$$

$$P(X \le 10) \approx P\left(Z \le \frac{10 - 25}{\sqrt{\dfrac{50^4}{100^2 \times 99}}}\right) = P(Z \le -5.9699) \approx 0$$

16. a) $\overline{X} = \sum\limits_{i=1}^{16} x_i/16$ where $X_i \sim N(\mu,4)$

$$\overline{X} \sim N(\mu,1/4)$$

$$P = P\,(\overline{X} \ge 5\,|H_0) = P\left(Z \ge \frac{5-4}{\sqrt{(1/4)}}\right) = P(Z \ge 2) =$$

$$= 0.0228$$

b) $P = 0.05$ corresponds to $z = 1.645$

$$\frac{\overline{X}_0 - 4}{1/2} = 1.645 \text{ gives } \overline{X}_0 = 4.82$$

17. a) $X \sim N(\mu, 1/4)$ (see the solution to Exercise 16)

$$
P = \begin{cases}
P\left(Z \leq \dfrac{5-\mu}{\sqrt{(1/4)}}\right) & \text{for } \mu > 5 \\[3mm]
P\left(Z \geq \dfrac{5-\mu}{\sqrt{(1/4)}}\right) & \text{otherwise}
\end{cases}
$$

Beneath is a table for the P-value function

P	0.001	0.023	0.159	0.500	0.159	0.023	0.001
μ	3.50	4.00	4.50	5.00	5.50	6.00	6.50

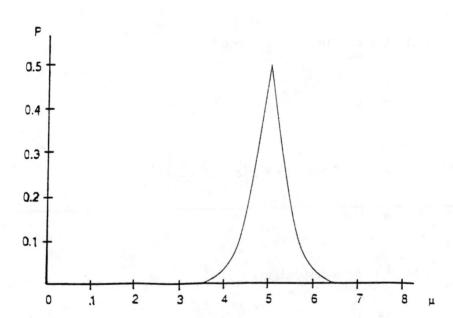

b) $P = 0.05$ for $\mu = 4.02$ and $\mu = 5.98$

18. $X \sim bin(10,CI)$

$$p(x) = \binom{n}{x} CI^x \, (1 - CI)^{n-x}$$

$$P = P \, (x \leq 1 \mid CI = 0.2) = \binom{10}{0} 0.2^0 \times 0.8^{10} +$$

$$+ \binom{10}{1} 0.2 \times 0.8^9 = 0.376$$

19. a) $X_1 \sim bin(100,CI_1)$

$X_2 \sim bin(100,CI_2)$

$\hat{RD} = \hat{CI_2} - \hat{CI_1}$

$$E(\hat{RD}) = E\left(\frac{X_2}{100}\right) - E\left(\frac{X_1}{100}\right) =$$

$$= CI_2 - CI_1$$

$$var(\hat{RD}) = var\left(\frac{X_2}{100}\right) + var\left(\frac{X_1}{100}\right) =$$

$$= \frac{CI_2 \ (1 - CI_2)}{100} + \frac{CI_1 \ (1 - CI_1)}{100}$$

Under H_0 is $var(\hat{RD}) = \frac{2}{100} CI(1 - CI)$

where CI is the common cumulative incidence.

$var(\hat{RD})$ can then be estimated as $\dfrac{2}{100} \times \dfrac{25}{200} \times \dfrac{175}{200}$

$$\hat{RD} \approx N\left(0, \frac{2}{100} \times \frac{25}{200} \times \frac{175}{200}\right)$$

$$P = P\left(Z \geq \frac{15/100 - 10/100}{\sqrt{\left(\frac{2}{100} \times \frac{25}{200} \times \frac{175}{200}\right)}}\right) = 0.143$$

b)

$$P = P\left(Z \geq \frac{A_1 - \frac{N_1 A}{N}}{\sqrt{\left(\frac{A \ (N - A) \ N_1 \ N_0}{N^2(N - 1)}\right)}}\right) =$$

$$= P\left(Z \geq \frac{15 - \frac{100 \times 25}{200}}{\sqrt{\left(\frac{25 \times 175 \times 100 \times 100}{200^2 \times 199}\right)}}\right) = 0.143$$

20. Let X_1 be the number of exposed in the first group. Given a certain total number of exposed, X_1 is hyper-geometrically distributed under the null hypothesis.

$$P = P(X_1 \geq 5) = \frac{\binom{5}{5}\binom{5}{4}}{\binom{10}{9}} = 1/2$$

21. $\mu_{L,U} = x_0 \pm 1.96 \sqrt{var(X)} =$

$$= 5 \pm 1.96 \sqrt{4} = 1.08,\ 8.92$$

22. Consider $\overline{X} = \dfrac{\sum\limits_{i=1}^{4} X_i}{4}$ where $X_i \sim N(\mu, 4)$

$\overline{X} \sim N(\mu, 1)$

$\mu_{L,U} = \overline{x}_0 \pm 1.96 \sqrt{var(\overline{X})} = 5 \pm 1.96 \times 1 =$

$$= 3.04,\ 6.96$$

23. $\hat{I} = A/R,\ A \sim$ Poisson $(I\ R)$

$E(\hat{I}) = 1/R\ (E(A)) = I$

$var(\hat{I}) = 1/R^2 \; var(A)$ and is estimated as A/R^2

$\hat{I} \sim N(I, A/R^2)$ for large materials

24. a) $A_0 = 20$

   Table 1 gives:

   $A_{L,U} = 12.217, 30.888$

   Division by 3000 gives

   $I_{L,U} = 0.00407, 0.0103$

   b) alternative 1

   $A \sim$ Poisson(μ), $A = 20$ is an estimation of μ

   Normal distribution approximation gives $A \sim N(20,20)$

   $\mu_{L,U} = A \pm 1.96 \sqrt{A} = 20 \pm 1.96 \sqrt{20} =$

   $= 11.23, 28.77$

   Division by 3000 gives $I_{L,U} = 0.00375, 0.00959$

   c) alternative 2

   $\hat{I} \sim N(I, A/R^2)$

$$I_{L,U} = A/R \pm 1.96 \sqrt{A/R^2} =$$

$$= \frac{20}{3,000} \pm 1.96 \sqrt{\frac{20}{3,000^2}} =$$

$$= 0.00375, \ 0.00959$$

25. $\hat{CI} = A/N$ where $A \sim bin\ (N,CI)$

$$E(\hat{CI}) = 1/N\ E(A) = CI$$

$$var(\hat{CI}) = 1/N^2\ var(A) = \frac{CI(1-CI)}{N}$$

The variance can be estimated as $\dfrac{A/N\ (1-A/N)}{N}$

$$\hat{CI} \sim N\left(CI,\ \frac{A/N\ (1-A/N)}{N}\right) \text{ when } N \text{ is large}$$

26.

$$CI_{L,U} = A/N \pm 1.96 \sqrt{\left(\frac{A/N(1-A/N)}{N}\right)} =$$

$$= \frac{100}{10000} \pm 1.96 \sqrt{\left(\frac{100/10000(1-100/10000)}{10000}\right)} =$$

$$= 0.00805, \ 0.0120$$

27. a)

$$CI_{L,U} = A/N \pm 1.96 \sqrt{\left(\frac{A/N(1 - A/N)}{N} \right)} =$$

$$= 6/6000 \pm 1.96 \sqrt{\left(\frac{6/6000(1 - 6/6000)}{6000} \right)} =$$

$$= 0.000200, \ 0.00180$$

b) $\hat{CI} = A/N, \ A \sim$ Poisson (6)

Table 1 gives $A_{L,U} = 2.202, \ 13.059$

Division by 6000 gives $CI_{L,U} = 0.000367, \ 0.00218$

28. a) $\hat{RD} = \hat{I}_1 - \hat{I}_0$

$$var \ (\hat{RD}) = A_1/R_1^2 + A_0/R_0^2$$

Normal distribution approximation gives:

$$RD_{L,U} = \hat{RD} \pm 1.96 \sqrt{var(\hat{RD})} =$$

$$= \frac{41}{28010} - \frac{15}{19017} \pm 1.96 \sqrt{\left(\frac{41}{28010^2} + \frac{15}{19017^2} \right)} =$$

$$= 7.49 \times 10^{-5}, \ 0.00128$$

b) $\ln\hat{RR} \sim N(\ln\hat{RR}, \ 1/A_1 + 1/A_0)$

$$RR_{L,U} = \exp\left(\ln\frac{41 \times 19017}{28010 \times 15} \pm 1.96\sqrt{\left(\frac{1}{41} + \frac{1}{15}\right)}\right) =$$

$$= 1.03, \ 3.35$$

c) $RR_{L,U} = \hat{R}R^{(1 \pm 1.96/Z)}$

$$z = \frac{\ln\hat{R}R - 0}{\sqrt{var(\ln\hat{R}R)}} = \frac{\ln\left(\dfrac{41 \times 19017}{28010 \times 15}\right)}{\sqrt{(1/41 + 1/15)}} = 2.049$$

$$RR_{L,U} = 1.03, \ 3.35$$

d) $A_1 \,|\, A \sim bin\left(A, \dfrac{R_1 I_1}{R_1 I_1 + R_0 I_0}\right)$

Normal distribution approximation gives:

$$A_1 \sim N\left(A\,\frac{R_1 I_1}{R_1 I_1 + R_0 I_0}, \ A\,\frac{R_1 I_1}{R_1 I_1 + R_0 I_0}\left(1 - \frac{R_1 I_1}{R_1 I_1 + R_0 I_0}\right)\right)$$

Under the null hypothesis is $I_1 = I_0$;

$$z = \frac{A_1 - A\,\dfrac{R_1}{R_1 + R_0}}{\sqrt{\left(A\,\dfrac{R_1}{R_1 + R_0}\,\dfrac{R_0}{R_1 + R_0}\right)}} = \frac{41 - 56\,\dfrac{28010}{47027}}{\sqrt{\left(56\,\dfrac{28010}{47027}\,\dfrac{19017}{47027}\right)}} =$$

$$= 2.082$$

$$RR_{L,U} = \hat{R}R^{(1 \pm 1.96/z)} =$$

$$= \left(\frac{41 \times 19017}{28010 \times 15}\right)^{1 \pm 1.96/2.082} =$$

$$= 1.04, \ 3.32$$

29. a) An approximate 95% confidence interval based on normal distribution approximation is calculated as:

$$RD_{L,U} = \hat{C}I_1 - \hat{C}I_0 \pm 1.96 \sqrt{\left(\frac{\hat{C}I_1(1 - \hat{C}I_1)}{N_1} + \frac{\hat{C}I_0(1 - \hat{C}I_0)}{N_0}\right)} =$$

$$= \frac{30}{204} - \frac{21}{205} \pm 1.96 \sqrt{\left(\frac{\dfrac{30}{204} \times \dfrac{174}{204}}{204} + \frac{\dfrac{21}{205} \times \dfrac{184}{205}}{205}\right)} =$$

$$= -0.0193, \ 0.109$$

b) $\ln(\hat{R}R) \sim N\left(\ln\hat{R}R, \ \dfrac{N_1 - A_1}{N_1 A_1} + \dfrac{N_0 - A_0}{N_0 A_0}\right)$

$$RR_{L,U} = \exp\left[\ln\left(\frac{30/204}{21/205}\right) \pm 1.96 \sqrt{\left(\frac{174}{204 \times 30} + \frac{184}{205 \times 21}\right)}\right] =$$

$$= 0.851, \ 2.42$$

c) Under the null hypothesis $RR = 1$ $A_1 | A$ is hypergeometrically distributed. Normal distribution approximation gives:

$$z = \frac{A_1 - \dfrac{AN_1}{N}}{\sqrt{\dfrac{A(N-A)N_1N_0}{N^2(N-1)}}} = \frac{30 - \dfrac{51 \times 204}{409}}{\sqrt{\dfrac{51 \times 358 \times 204 \times 205}{409^2 \times 408}}} = 1.364$$

$$RR_{L,U} = \hat{R}R^{(1 \pm 1.96/z)} = \left(\frac{30/204}{21/205}\right)^{(1 \pm 1.96/1.364)} =$$

$$= 0.854, \ 2.41$$

30. a) $OR_{L,U} = \exp[\ln \hat{O}R \pm 1.96 \sqrt{var(\ln \hat{O}R)}\ ] =$

$$= \exp\left(\ln \frac{ad}{bc} \pm 1.96 \sqrt{\left(\frac{1}{a} + \frac{1}{b} + \frac{1}{c} + \frac{1}{d}\right)}\right) =$$

$$= \exp\left(\ln \frac{96 \times 666}{104 \times 109} \pm \sqrt{\left(\frac{1}{96} + \frac{1}{104} + \frac{1}{109} + \frac{1}{666}\right)}\right) =$$

$$= 4.00, \ 7.95$$

b) Normal distribution approximation of the hyper-geometrical distribution gives:

$$z = \frac{a - \dfrac{M_1N_1}{T}}{\sqrt{\dfrac{M_1M_0N_1N_0}{T^2(T-1)}}} = \frac{96 - \dfrac{205 \times 200}{975}}{\sqrt{\dfrac{205 \times 770 \times 200 \times 775}{975^2 \times 974}}} =$$

$$= 10.50$$

$$OR_{L,U} = \hat{OR}^{(1 \pm 1.96/z)} =$$

$$= \left(\frac{96 \times 666}{104 \times 109} \right)^{(1 \pm 1.96/10.50)} = 4.08, \, 7.79$$

31. a) $\hat{RD}_{pool} = \dfrac{\sum w_i \, \hat{RD}_i}{\sum w_i}$

$$w_i = \left(\frac{A_{1i}}{R_{1i}^2} + \frac{A_{0i}}{R_{0i}^2} \right)^{-1}$$

$$w_1 = \frac{1}{\dfrac{32}{52407^2} + \dfrac{2}{18790^2}} = 5.775 \times 10^7$$

$$w_2 = \frac{1}{\dfrac{104}{43248^2} + \dfrac{12}{10673^2}} = 6.213 \times 10^6$$

$$\hat{RD}_{pool} = \frac{5.775 \times 10^7 \left(\dfrac{32}{52407} - \dfrac{2}{18790} \right) + 6.213 \times 10^6 \left(\dfrac{104}{43248} - \dfrac{12}{10673} \right)}{5.775 \times 10^7 + 6.213 \times 10^6} =$$

$$= 5.796 \times 10^{-4}$$

$$var(\hat{RD}_{pool}) = \frac{1}{\sum w_i}$$

$$RD_{pool,L,U} = \hat{R}D_{pool} \pm 1.96\sqrt{(1/\Sigma\ w_i)} =$$

$$= 5.796 \times 10^{-4} \pm 1.96 \sqrt{\frac{1}{5.775 \times 10^7 + 6.213 \times 10^6}} =$$

$$= 3.35 \times 10^{-4},\ 8.25 \times 10^{-4}$$

b) $\hat{R}R_1 = \dfrac{32/52407}{2/18790} = 5.737$ $\hat{R}R_2 = \dfrac{104/43248}{12/10673} = 2.139$

$$RR_{i,UG,\acute{O}G} = \exp\left(\ln\hat{R}R_i \pm 1.96 \sqrt{\left(\frac{1}{A_{1i}} + \frac{1}{A_{0i}}\right)}\right)$$

$$RR_{1,L,U} = \exp\left[\ln 5.737 \pm 1.96 \sqrt{(1/32 + 1/2)}\right] =$$
$$= 1.38,\ 23.9$$

$$RR_{2,L,U} = \exp\left[\ln 2.139 \pm 1.96 \sqrt{(1/104 + 1/12)}\right] =$$
$$= 1.18,\ 3.89$$

c) $\ln\hat{R}R_{pool} = \dfrac{\Sigma w_i\ \ln\hat{R}R_i}{\Sigma w_i}$

$$w_i = \frac{1}{var(\ln \hat{R}R_i)} \approx \frac{1}{1/A_{1i} + 1/A_{0i}}$$

$$w_1 = (1/32 + 1/2)^{-1} = 1.882$$

$$w_2 = (1/104 + 1/12)^{-1} = 10.76$$

$$\hat{RR}_{pool} = \exp\left(\frac{1.882 \ \ln\left(\dfrac{32/52407}{2/18790}\right) + 10.76 \ \ln\left(\dfrac{104/43248}{12/10673}\right)}{1.882 + 10.76}\right) =$$

$$= 2.477$$

$$RR_{pool,L,U} = \exp\ [\ln\hat{RR}_{pool} \pm 1.96\ \sqrt{(1/\Sigma\ w_i)}] =$$

$$= \exp\ [\ln\ 2.477 \pm 1.96\ \sqrt{(1.882 + 10.76)^{-1}}\ ] =$$

$$= 1.43,\ 4.30$$

d)
$$\hat{RR}_{MH} = \frac{\Sigma\ A_{1i}\ R_{0i}/R_i}{\Sigma\ A_{0i}\ R_{1i}/R_i} =$$

$$= \frac{\dfrac{32 \times 18790}{71197} + \dfrac{104 \times 10673}{53921}}{\dfrac{2 \times 52407}{71197} + \dfrac{12 \times 43248}{53921}} = 2.616$$

Normal distribution approximation based on a conditional analysis gives:

$$z = \frac{\sum A_{1i} - \sum \frac{A_i R_{1i}}{R_i}}{\sqrt{\left(\sum A_i \frac{R_{1i}}{R_i} \left(1 - \frac{R_{1i}}{R_i}\right)\right)}} =$$

$$= \frac{32 + 104 - \left(\frac{34 \times 52407}{71197} + \frac{116 \times 43248}{53921}\right)}{\sqrt{\left(\frac{34 \times 52407 \times 18790}{71197^2} + \frac{116 \times 43248 \times 10673}{53921^2}\right)}} =$$

$$= 3.585$$

$$RR_{MH,L,U} = \hat{R}R_{MH}^{(1 \pm 1.96/z)} =$$

$$= 2.616^{(1 \pm 1.96/3.585)} =$$

$$= 1.55, 4.43$$

e) $RR_{MH,L,U} = \exp\left[\ln\hat{R}R_{MH} \pm 1.96 \sqrt{var(\ln\hat{R}R_{pool})}\right] =$

$$= \exp\left(\ln 2.616 \pm 1.96 \sqrt{\frac{1}{1.882 + 10.76}}\right) =$$

$$= 1.51, 4.55$$

f)

$$var(\ln\hat{R}R_{MH}) \approx \frac{\sum A_i \, R_{1i} \, R_{0i}/R_i^2}{(\sum A_{1i} \, R_{0i}/R_i) \, (\sum A_{0i} R_{1i}/R_i)} =$$

$$= \frac{\dfrac{34 \times 52407 \times 18790}{71197^2} + \dfrac{116 \times 43248 \times 10673}{53921^2}}{\left(\dfrac{32 \times 18790}{71197} + \dfrac{104 \times 10673}{53921}\right)\left(\dfrac{2 \times 52407}{71197} + \dfrac{12 \times 43248}{53921}\right)} =$$

$$= 0.07767$$

$$RR_{MH,L,U} = \exp\left(\ln\hat{R}R_{MH} \pm 1.96 \sqrt{var(\ln\hat{R}R_{MH})}\;\right) =$$

$$= \exp\left(\ln 2.616 \pm 1.96 \sqrt{0.07767}\,\right) =$$

$$= 1.52, \; 4.52$$

32. a) $\hat{R}D_{pool} = \dfrac{\sum w_i \, \hat{R}D_i}{\sum w_i}$

$$w_i = \frac{1}{var(\hat{R}D_i)} \approx \left(\frac{\hat{C}I_{1i}(1-\hat{C}I_{1i})}{N_{1i}} + \frac{\hat{C}I_{0i}(1-\hat{C}I_{0i})}{N_{0i}}\right)^{-1}$$

$$w_1 = \left(\frac{8/106 \, (1-(8/106))}{106} + \frac{5/120 \, (1-(5/120))}{120}\right)^{-1} =$$

$$= 1009$$

$$w_2 = \left(\frac{22/98 \, (1-(22/98))}{98} + \frac{16/85 \, (1-(16/85))}{85}\right)^{-1} =$$

$$= 279.8$$

$$\hat{R}D_{pool} = \frac{1009(8/106 - 5/120) + 279.8(22/98 - 16/85)}{1009 + 279.8} =$$

$$= 0.03434$$

$$RD_{pool,L,U} = \hat{R}D_{pool} \pm 1.96 \sqrt{(1/\Sigma\, w_i)} =$$

$$= 0.03434 \pm 1.96 \sqrt{\frac{1}{1009 + 279.8}} =$$

$$= -0.0203,\ 0.0889$$

b) $\hat{R}R_1 = \dfrac{8/106}{5/120} = 1.811$ $\hat{R}R_2 = \dfrac{22/98}{16/85} = 1.193$

$$RR_{i,L,U} = \exp\left(\ln\hat{R}R_i \pm 1.96 \sqrt{\left(\frac{N_{1i} - A_{1i}}{N_{1i}\, A_{1i}} + \frac{N_{0i} - A_{0i}}{N_{0i}\, A_{0i}}\right)}\right)$$

$$RR_{1,L,U} = \exp\left(\ln 1.811 \pm 1.96 \sqrt{\left(\frac{106 - 8}{106 \times 8} + \frac{120 - 5}{120 \times 5}\right)}\right) =$$

$$= 0.611,\ 5.37$$

$$RR_{2,L,U} = \exp\left(\ln 1.193 \pm \sqrt{\left(\frac{98 - 22}{98 \times 22} + \frac{85 - 16}{85 \times 16}\right)}\right) =$$

$$= 0.671,\ 2.12$$

c) $\ln\hat{R}R_{pool} = \dfrac{\Sigma w_i \ln\hat{R}R_i}{\Sigma w_i}$

$w_i = \dfrac{1}{var(\ln\hat{R}R_i)} \approx \left(\dfrac{N_{1i} - A_{1i}}{N_{1i} A_{1i}} + \dfrac{N_{0i} - A_{0i}}{N_{0i} A_{0i}} \right)^{-1}$

$w_1 = \left(\dfrac{106 - 8}{106 \times 8} + \dfrac{120 - 5}{120 \times 5} \right)^{-1} = 3.255$

$w_2 = \left(\dfrac{98 - 22}{98 \times 22} + \dfrac{85 - 16}{85 \times 16} \right)^{-1} = 11.63$

$\hat{R}R_{pool} = \exp\left(\dfrac{3.255 \ln 1.811 + 11.63 \ln 1.193}{3.255 + 11.63} \right) =$

$= 1.307$

$RR_{pool,L,U} = \exp(\ln\hat{R}R_{pool} \pm 1.96 \sqrt{(1/\Sigma w_i)}) =$

$= \exp(\ln 1.307 \pm 1.96 \sqrt{(3.255 + 11.63)^{-1}}) =$

$= 0.786,\ 2.17$

d)

$\hat{R}R_{MH} = \dfrac{\Sigma A_{1i} N_{0i}/N_i}{\Sigma A_{0i} N_{1i}/N_i} =$

$= \dfrac{8 \times 120/226 + 22 \times 85/183}{5 \times 106/226 + 16 \times 98/183} = 1.326$

Normal distribution approximation based on a conditional analysis gives:

$$z = \frac{\sum A_{1i} - \sum \dfrac{A_i \, N_{1i}}{N_i}}{\sqrt{\sum \dfrac{A_i \, (N_i - A_i) \, N_{1i} \, N_{0i}}{N_i^2 \, (N_i - 1)}}} =$$

$$= \frac{22 + 8 - (13 \times 106/226 + 38 \times 98/183)}{\sqrt{\left(\dfrac{13 \times 213 \times 106 \times 120}{226^2 \times 225} + \dfrac{38 \times 145 \times 98 \times 85}{183^2 \times 182} \right)}} =$$

$$= 1.092$$

$$RR_{MH,L,U} = \hat{R}R_{MH}^{(1 \pm 1.96/z)} =$$

$$= 1.326^{(1 \pm 1.96/1.092)} =$$

$$= 0.799, \ 2.20$$

e) $RR_{MH,L,U} = \exp \left[\ln\hat{R}R_{MH} \pm 1.96 \sqrt{var(\ln\hat{R}R_{pool})} \, \right] =$

$$= \exp \left(\ln 1.326 \pm 1.96 \sqrt{(3.255 + 11.63)^{-1}} \right. =$$

$$= 0.800, \ 2.21$$

f)

$$var(\ln\hat{R}R_{MH}) \approx \frac{\sum (A_i N_{1i} N_{0i} - A_{1i} A_{0i} N_i)/N_i^2}{(\sum A_{1i} N_{0i}/N_i) \, (\sum A_{0i} N_{1i}/N_i)} =$$

$$= \frac{\dfrac{13 \times 106 \times 120 - 8 \times 5 \times 226}{226^2} + \dfrac{38 \times 98 \times 85 - 22 \times 16 \times 183}{183^2}}{\left(\dfrac{8 \times 120}{226} + \dfrac{22 \times 85}{183} \right) \left(\dfrac{5 \times 106}{226} + \dfrac{16 \times 98}{183} \right)} =$$

$$= 0.06707$$

$$RR_{MH,L,U} = \exp\,(\ln\hat{R}R_{MH} \pm 1.96\,\sqrt{var(\ln\hat{R}R_{MH})}\,) =$$

$$= \exp\,(\ln\,1.326 \pm 1.96\,\sqrt{0.06707}\,) =$$

$$= 0.798,\ 2.20$$

33. a) $\hat{O}R_1 = \dfrac{15 \times 1409}{64 \times 319} = 1.035$ $\hat{O}R_2 = \dfrac{8 \times 381}{72 \times 53} = 0.7987$

$$OR_{i,L,U} = \exp\,(\ln\hat{O}R_i \pm 1.96\,\sqrt{(1/a_i + 1/b_i + 1/c_i + 1/d_i)}\,)$$

$$OR_{1,L,U} = \exp\,(\ln\,1.035 \pm 1.96\,\sqrt{(1/15 + 1/64 + 1/319 + 1/1409)}\,) =$$

$$= 0.582,\ 1.84$$

$$OR_{2,L,U} = \exp\,(\ln\,0.7987 \pm 1.96\,\sqrt{(1/8 + 1/72 + 1/53 + 1/381)}\,) =$$

$$= 0.364,\ 1.75$$

b) $\ln\hat{O}R_{pool} = \dfrac{\Sigma\,w_i\,\ln\hat{O}R_i}{\Sigma\,w_i}$

$$w_i = \dfrac{1}{var(\ln\hat{O}R_i)} \approx \dfrac{1}{1/a_i + 1/b_i + 1/c_i + 1/d_i}$$

$$w_1 = (1/15 + 1/64 + 1/319 + 1/1409)^{-1} = 11.61$$

$$w_2 = (1/8 + 1/72 + 1/53 + 1/381)^{-1} = 6.235$$

$$\hat{OR}_{pool} = \exp\left(\frac{11.61 \ \ln 1.035 + 6.235 \ \ln 0.7987}{11.61 + 6.235}\right) =$$

$$= 0.9455$$

$$OR_{pool,L,U} = \exp(\ln\hat{OR}_{pool} \pm 1.96 \sqrt{(1/\Sigma \ w_i)}) =$$

$$= \exp (\ln 0.9455 \pm 1.96 \sqrt{(11.61 + 6.235)^{-1}} \ ) =$$

$$= 0.595, \ 1.50$$

c) $$\hat{OR}_{MH} = \frac{\Sigma \ a_i d_i /T_i}{\Sigma \ b_i c_i /T_i}$$

$$\hat{OR}_{MH} = \frac{\dfrac{15 \times 1409}{1807} + \dfrac{8 \times 381}{514}}{\dfrac{64 \times 319}{1807} + \dfrac{72 \times 53}{514}} = 0.9415$$

Normal distribution approximation based on a conditional analysis gives:

$$z = \frac{\Sigma \ a_i - \Sigma \ N_{1i} M_{1i}/T_i}{\sqrt{\Sigma \ \dfrac{N_{1i} N_{0i} M_{1i} M_{0i}}{T_i^2 (T_i - 1)}}} =$$

$$= \frac{15 + 8 - \left(\dfrac{79 \times 334}{1807} + \dfrac{80 \times 61}{514}\right)}{\sqrt{\left(\dfrac{79 \times 1728 \times 334 \times 1473}{1807^2 \times 1806} + \dfrac{80 \times 434 \times 61 \times 453}{514^2 \times 513}\right)}} =$$

$$= -0.2551$$

$$OR_{MH,L,U} = \hat{O}R_{MH}^{(1 \pm 1.96/z)} = 0.9415^{(1 \pm 1.96/-0.2551)} =$$

$$= 0.592, \ 1.50$$

34. a) $\hat{O}R_1 = \dfrac{10 \times 95}{90 \times 5} = 2.111$

$\hat{O}R_2 = \dfrac{3 \times 50}{47 \times 0} = ?$ Undefined

$$OR_{i,L,U} = \exp(\ln\hat{O}R_i \pm 1.96\sqrt{(1/a_i + 1/b_i + 1/c_i + 1/d_i)}\,) =$$

$$OR_{1,L,U} = \exp(\ln 2.111 \pm 1.96\sqrt{(1/10 + 1/90 + 1/5 + 1/95)}\,) =$$

$$= 0.694, \ 6.41$$

Neither can $OR_{2,L,U}$ be calculated.

b) $\ln\hat{O}R_{pool} = \dfrac{\Sigma \ w_i \ \ln\hat{O}R_i}{\Sigma \ w_i}$

$$w_i = \dfrac{1}{var(\ln\hat{O}R_i)} \approx \dfrac{1}{1/a_i + 1/b_i + 1/c_i + 1/d_i}$$

$w_1 = (1/10 + 1/90 + 1/5 + 1/95)^{-1} = 3.109$

w_2 undefined when any cell frequency = 0

This means that a pooled analysis is unsuitable when strata contain one or more zeros.

c)

$$\hat{O}R_{MH} = \frac{\sum a_i d_i / T_i}{\sum b_i c_i / T_i} =$$

$$= \frac{10 \times 95/200 + 3 \times 50/100}{90 \times 5/200 + 47 \times 0/100} = 2.778$$

$$z = \frac{\sum a_i - \sum N_{1i} M_{1i} / T_i}{\sqrt{\left(\dfrac{N_{1i} N_{0i} M_{1i} M_{0i}}{T_i^2 (T_i - 1)} \right)}} =$$

$$= \frac{10 + 3 - (100 \times 15/200 + 50 \times 3/100)}{\sqrt{\left(\dfrac{100 \times 100 \times 15 \times 185}{200^2 \times 199} + \dfrac{50 \times 50 \times 3 \times 97}{100^2 \times 99} \right)}} =$$

$$= 1.947$$

$$OR_{MH,L,U} = O\hat{R}_{MH}^{(1 \pm 1.96/z)} =$$

$$= 2.778^{(1 \pm 1.96/1.947)} =$$

$$= 0.993,\ 7.77$$

d) $$var(\ln \hat{O}R_{MH}) \approx \frac{\sum \left(\dfrac{a_i + d_i}{T_i} \right) \left(\dfrac{a_i d_i}{T_i} \right)}{2 \left(\sum \dfrac{a_i d_i}{T_i} \right)^2} +$$

$$+\ \frac{\sum\left(\left(\dfrac{a_i + d_i}{T_i}\right)\left(\dfrac{b_i\ c_i}{T_i}\right) + \left(\dfrac{b_i + c_i}{T_i}\right)\left(\dfrac{a_i\ d_i}{T_i}\right)\right)}{2\ \sum\dfrac{a_i\ d_i}{T_i}\ \sum\dfrac{b_i\ c_i}{T_i}}\ +$$

$$+\ \frac{\sum\left(\dfrac{b_i + c_i}{T_i}\right)\left(\dfrac{b_i\ c_i}{T_i}\right)}{2\left(\sum\dfrac{b_i\ c_i}{T_i}\right)^2}\ =$$

$$=\ \frac{\left(\dfrac{10 + 95}{200}\right)\left(\dfrac{10 \times 95}{200}\right) + \left(\dfrac{3 + 50}{100}\right)\left(\dfrac{3 \times 50}{100}\right)}{2\left(\dfrac{10 \times 95}{200} + \dfrac{3 \times 50}{100}\right)^2}\ +$$

$$+\ \frac{\left(\left(\dfrac{10 + 95}{200}\right)\left(\dfrac{90 \times 5}{200}\right) + \left(\dfrac{90 + 5}{200}\right)\left(\dfrac{10 \times 95}{200}\right)\right) + \left(\left(\dfrac{3 + 50}{100}\right)\left(\dfrac{47 \times 0}{100}\right) + \left(\dfrac{47 + 0}{100}\right)\left(\dfrac{3 \times 50}{100}\right)\right)}{2\left(\dfrac{10 \times 95}{200} + \dfrac{3 \times 50}{100}\right)\left(\dfrac{90 \times 5}{200} + \dfrac{47 \times 0}{100}\right)}\ +$$

$$+\ \frac{\left(\dfrac{90 + 5}{200}\right)\left(\dfrac{90 \times 5}{200}\right) + \left(\dfrac{47 + 0}{100}\right)\left(\dfrac{47 \times 0}{100}\right)}{2\left(\dfrac{90 \times 5}{200} + \dfrac{47 \times 0}{100}\right)^2}\ =\ 0.2338$$

$$OR_{MH,L,U} = \exp(\ln\hat{O}R_{MH} \pm 1.96\ \sqrt{var(\ln\hat{O}R_{MH})}) =$$

$$= \exp(\ln 2.778 \pm 1.96\ \sqrt{0.2338}) =$$

$$= 1.08,\ 7.17$$

35. The Mantel-Haenszel estimator is simplified to:

$$\hat{O}R_{MH} = \frac{s}{t} = \frac{5}{1} = 5$$

The Mantel-Haenszel test is simplified to:

$$z = \frac{s - t}{\sqrt{(s + t)}} = \frac{5 - 1}{\sqrt{(5 + 1)}} = 1.633$$

$$OR_{MH,L,U} = \hat{O}R_{MH}^{(1 \pm 1.96/z)} =$$

$$= 5^{(1 \pm 1.96/1.633)} =$$

$$= 0.725, \ 34.5$$

36. a)
$$S\hat{R}R = \frac{\Sigma v_i \hat{I}_{1i}}{\Sigma v_i \hat{I}_{0i}} = \frac{1/10 \times 0.010 + 9/10 \times 0.030}{1/10 \times 0.005 + 9/10 \times 0.025} =$$

$$= \frac{0.02800}{0.02300} = 1.217$$

b)
$$var(\ln S\hat{R}R) \approx \frac{\Sigma v_i^2 A_{1i}/R_{1i}^2}{[\Sigma v_i \hat{I}_{1i}]^2} + \frac{\Sigma v_i^2 A_{0i}/R_{0i}^2}{[\Sigma v_i \hat{I}_{0i}]^2} =$$

$$= \frac{(1/10)^2 \times 30/3000^2 + (9/10)^2 \times 30/1000^2}{0.028^2} +$$

$$+ \frac{(1/10)^2 \times 5/1000^2 + (9/10)^2 \times 225/9000^2}{0.023^2} =$$

$$= 0.03529$$

$$SRR_{L,U} = \exp\ (\ln\ 1.217 \pm 1.96\sqrt{0.03529}\ ) = 0.842,\ 1.76$$

c) The choice of weights influences the point estimate as well as the precision.

37. $S\hat{M}R = O/E$

$O \sim$ Poisson; Table 1 gives

$O_{L,U} = 0.619,\ 8.767$

Division by $E = 1.5$ gives $SMR_{L,U} = 0.413,\ 5.85$

38. $O \sim$ Poisson $(SMR \times E)$

$E(O) = SMR \times E = O$

$var(O) = SMR \times E = O$

$O \sim N(O,O)$

$O_{L,U} = O \pm 1.96\sqrt{O}\ = \pm\ 1.96\sqrt{30}\ = 19.26,\ 40.74$

Division by $E = 25$ gives $SMR_{L,U} = 0.771, 1.63$

39. a) $\hat{S}MR = O/E$

$O = 120$

$E = \sum R_{1i} I_{0i} = 6000 \times 0.005 + 2000 \times 0.025 = 80.00$

$SMR = \dfrac{120}{80.00} = 1.500$

In order to calculate z, for example, the Mantel-Haenszel analogy regarding cohort studies with incidence data can be used.

$$z = \frac{A_1 - E(A_i)}{\sqrt{(\text{var}(A_1))}} = \frac{\sum A_{1i} - \sum \dfrac{A_i R_{1i}}{R_i}}{\sqrt{\left(\sum A_i \dfrac{R_{1i}}{R_i} \left(1 - \dfrac{R_{1i}}{R_i} \right) \right)}} =$$

$$= \frac{120 - \left(\dfrac{65 \times 6000}{7000} + \dfrac{285 \times 2000}{11000} \right)}{\sqrt{\left(65 \times \dfrac{6000 \times 1000}{7000^2} + 285 \dfrac{2000 \times 9000}{11000^2} \right)}} =$$

$= 1.757$

$SMR_{L,U} = \hat{S}MR^{(1 \pm 1.96/z)} =$

$= 1.500^{(1 \pm 1.96/1.757)} =$

$= 0.954, 2.36$

b) $S\hat{M}R = O/E$

$E(S\hat{M}R) = E(O/E) = O/E$

$var(S\hat{M}R) = var(O/E) = O/E^2$

$S\hat{M}R \sim N(S\hat{M}R, S\hat{M}R/E)$

$SMR_{L,U} = S\hat{M}R \pm 1.96\sqrt{S\hat{M}R/E}$ =

= $1.500 \pm 1.96\sqrt{(1.500/80.00)}$ =

= $1.23, 1.77$

c) $S\hat{M}R = O/E$

$E(\ln S\hat{M}R) \approx \ln S\hat{M}R$

$var(\ln S\hat{M}R) = var(\ln(O/E)) \approx \dfrac{1}{(O/E)^2} var(O/E)$ =

$= \dfrac{E^2}{O^2}\, \dfrac{O}{E^2} = \dfrac{1}{O}$

$SMR_{L,U} = \exp(\ln S\hat{M}R \pm 1.96\sqrt{var(\ln S\hat{M}R)})$ =

= $\exp(\ln 1.500 \pm 1.96\sqrt{(1/120)}$ =

= $1.25, 1.79$

d) $\quad S\hat{M}R = \dfrac{\Sigma\ v_i\ \hat{I}_{1i}}{\Sigma\ v_i\ \hat{I}_{0i}}$

Where v_i is achieved from the exposed population.

Let $v_i = R_{1i}$

$$var(\ln S\hat{M}R) \approx \frac{\Sigma v_i^2\ A_{1i}/R_{1i}^2}{(\Sigma v_i \hat{I}_{1i})^2} + \frac{\Sigma v_i^2\ A_{0i}/R_{0i}^2}{(\Sigma v_i \hat{I}_{0i})^2} =$$

$$= \frac{\Sigma A_{1i}}{(\Sigma A_{1i})^2} + \frac{\Sigma R_{1i}^2\ A_{0i}/R_{0i}^2}{(\Sigma R_{1i}\ A_{0i}/R_{0i})^2} =$$

$$= \frac{1}{120} + \frac{6000^2 \times 5/1000^2 + 2000^2 \times 225/9000^2}{(6000 \times 5/1000 + 2000 \times 225/9000)^2} =$$

$$= 0.03819$$

$SMR_{L,U} = \exp(\ln S\hat{M}R \pm 1.96\ \sqrt{var(\ln S\hat{M}R)}) =$

$= \exp(\ln 1.500 \pm 1.96\ \sqrt{0.03819}) =$

$= 1.02,\ 2.20$

e)

$$\hat{R}R_{MH} = \frac{\Sigma\ A_{1i}\ R_{0i}\ /\ R_i}{\Sigma\ A_{0i}\ R_{1i}\ /\ R_i} =$$

$$= \frac{60 \times 1000/7000 + 60 \times 9000/11000}{5 \times 6000/7000 + 225 \times 2000/11000} =$$

$$= 1.276$$

According to 39a $z = 1.757$

$$RR_{MH,L,U} = \hat{R}R_{MH}^{(1 \pm 1.96/z)} =$$

$$= 1.276^{(1 \pm 1.96/1.757)} =$$

$$= 0.972, \ 1.68$$

f) The differences primarily depend on the fact that in Exercises a, d, and e, unlike Exercises b and c, the random error in the reference group is taken into account.

40. a) $\hat{\mu} = x$

$$E(\hat{\mu}) = E(X) = \mu$$

$$var(\hat{\mu}) = var(X) = \mu$$

b) The probability function for X is

$$p(x) = e^{-\mu} \ \mu^x/x! \ = L(\mu)$$

$$\ln L = -\mu + x \ln \mu - \ln x!$$

Derivation on μ gives

$$\frac{dL}{d\mu} = -1 + \frac{x}{\mu}$$

$$\frac{dL}{d\mu} = 0 \text{ gives } \mu = x$$

REFERENCES

Ahlbom A & Norell S. *Introduction to Modern Epidemiology.* Chestnut Hill, MA: Epidemiology Resources Inc., 1990.

Armitage P. *Statistical methods in medical research.* Oxford London Edinburgh Melbourne: Blackwell Scientific Publishers, 1971.

Breslow NE. Elementary methods of cohort analysis. *International Journal of Epidemiology* 1984;13:112-115.

Breslow NE & Day NE. Indirect standardization and multiplicative models for rates, with reference to age adjustment of cancer incidence and relative frequency data. *Journal of Chronic Diseases* 1975;28:289-303.

Breslow NE & Day NE. *Statistical methods in cancer research, Vol. 1.* The analysis of case-control studies. International Agency for Research on Cancer, Lyon 1980.

Breslow NE & Day NE. *Statistical methods in cancer research,* Vol. 2. The analysis of cohort studies. International Agency for Research on Cancer, Lyon 1987.

Breslow NE & Liang KY. The variance of the Mantel-Haenszel estimator. *Biometrics* 1982;38:943-952.

Breslow NE, Lubin JH, Marek P & Langholz. Multiplicative models and cohort analysis. *Journal of the American Statistical Association* 1983;78:1-12.

Breslow N & Powers W. Are there two logistic regressions for retrospective studies? *Biometrics* 1978;34:100-105.

Cole P. The evolving case-control study. *Journal of Chronic Diseases* 1979;32:15-27.

Colton T. *Statistics in Medicine.* Boston: Little, Brown and Company, 1974.

Cornfield JA. A statistical problem arising from retrospective studies. In Neyman J (ed.): *Proceedings Third Berkeley Symposium, Vol. 4.* Berkeley: University of California Press, 1956:135-148.

Cox DR. Regression models and life tables. *Journal of the Royal Statistical Society. Series B* 1972;187-220.

Elandt-Johnson RC. Definition of rates: Some remarks of their use and misuse. *American Journal of Epidemiology* 1975;102:267-271.

Epidemiology Monitor 1987;8: Inventory of free or inexpensive IBM-PC compatible software for epidemiologists.

Fisz M. *Probability theory and mathematical statistics.* New York, London, Sydney: John Wiley and Sons, 1963.

Freiman J, Chalmers TC, Smith H Jr. & Kuebler RR. The importance of beta, the type II error and sample size in the design and interpretation of the randomized control trial: survey of 71 "negative" trials. *New England Journal of Medicine* 1978;299:690-694.

Gart JJ. Point and interval estimation of the common odds ratio in the combination of 2 x 2 tables with fixed marginals. *Biometrika* 1970;57:471-475.

Gart JJ. Statistical analyses of the relative risk. *Environmental Health Perspectives* 1979;32:157-167.

Gleick J. Chaos. *Making a new science.* Viking Penguin Inc., 1987.

Greenland S. Limitations of the logistic analysis of epidemiologic data. *American Journal of Epidemiology* 1979;110:693-698.

Greenland S. A counterexample to the test-based principle of setting confidence limits. *American Journal of Epidemiology* 1984;120:4-7.

Greenland S. Quantitative methods in the review of epidemiologic literature. *Epidemiologic reviews* 1987;9:1-30.

Greenland S & Robins JM. Estimation of a common effect parameter from sparse follow-up data. *Biometrics* 1985;41:55-68.

Guilbaud O. On the large sample distribution of the Mantel-Haenszel odds-ratio estimator. *Biometrics* 1983;39:523-525.

Halperin M. Re: "Estimability and estimation in case-referent studies." Letter to the Editor. *American Journal of Epidemiology* 1977;105:496-498.

Hill AB. The environment and disease: Association or causation? *Proceedings of the Royal Society of Medicine* 1965;58:295-300.

Hill AB. Principles of medical statistics. *The Lancet Limited* 1967.

Hoem JM. The statistical theory of demographic rates. *Scandinavian Journal of Statistics* 1976;3:169-185.

Hoem JM. Statistical analysis of a multiplicative model and its application to the standardization of vital rates. *International Statistical Reviews* 1987;55:119-152.

Hoem JM & Ahlbom A. Statistical analysis of multiplicative models and its application to the standardization of vital rates. Part I. Consistency aspects. Laboratory of Actuarial Mathematics, University of Copenhagen 1979.

Mantel N. Chi-square tests with one degree of freedom: Extensions of the Mantel-Haenszel procedure. *Journal of the American Statistical Association* 1963;58:690-700.

Mantel N, Brown C, Byar DP. Tests for homogeneity of effect in an epidemiologic investigation. *American Journal of Epidemiology* 1977;106:125-129.

Mantel N & Haenszel W. Statistical aspects of the analysis of data from retrospective studies of disease. *Journal of the National Cancer Institute* 1959;22:719-749.

Miettinen OS. Confounding and effect-modification. *American Journal of Epidemiology* 1974;100:350-353.

Miettinen OS. Estimability and estimation in case-referent studies. *American Journal of Epidemiology* 1976;103:226-235.

Miettinen OS. Theoretical epidemiology. Principles of occurrence research in medicine. New York: John Wiley & Sons, 1985.

Miettinen OS & Nurminen M. Comparative analysis of two rates. *Statistics in Medicine* 1985;4:213-226.

Norell SE. A short course in epidemiology. New York: Raven Press, 1991.

Nurminen M. Analysis of epidemiologic case-base studies for binary data. Manuscript.

Oaks M. *Statistical inference: A commentary for the social and behavioral sciences.* Chichester: John Wiley and Sons, 1986.

Poole C. Beyond the confidence interval. *American Journal of Public Health* 1987;77:195-199.

Robins JM, Greenland S & Breslow NE. A general estimator for the variance of the Mantel-Haenszel odds ratio. *American Journal of Epidemiology* 1986;124:719-723.

Rothman KJ. Synergy and antagonism in cause-effect relationships. *American Journal of Epidemiology* 1974;99:385-388.

Rothman KJ. Estimation of synergy or antagonism. *American Journal of Epidemiology* 1976;103:506-511.

Rothman KJ. Causes. *American Journal of Epidemiology* 1976;104:587-592.

Rothman KJ. A show of confidence. *New England Journal of Medicine* 1978; 299:1362-1363.

Rothman KJ. *Modern epidemiology*. Boston: Little, Brown and Company, 1986.

Rothman KJ. No adjustments are needed for multiple comparisons. *Epidemiology* 1990;1:43-46.

Rothman KJ & Boice JD Jr. Epidemiologic analysis with a programmable calculator. Chestnut Hill, MA: Epidemiology Resources Inc., 1982.

Rothman KJ, Greenland S & Walker AM. Concepts of interaction. *American Journal of Epidemiology* 1980;99:385-388.

Scheffe H. *The analysis of variance*. Wiley, New York 1959.

Scherg H. Chance significances in case-control studies when using a long questionnaire. *Meth Inform Med* 1980;19:215-219.

Sverdrup E. Significance testing in multiple statistical inference. *Scandinavian Journal of Statistics* 1976;3:73-77.

Tarone RE. On summary estimators of relative risk. *Journal of Chronic Diseases* 1981;34:463-468.

Thomas D, Siemiatycki J, Dewar R, Robins J, Goldberg M & Armstrong BG. The problem of multiple inference in studies designed to generate hypotheses. *American Journal of Epidemiology* 1985;122:1080-1092.

Walker AM. Proportion of disease attributable to the combined effect of two factors. *International Journal of Epidemiology* 1981;10:81-85.

Walker AM. Reporting results of epidemiologic studies. *American Journal of Public Health* 1986;76:556-58.

Walker SH & Duncan DB. Estimation of the probability of an event as a function of several variables. *Biometrika* 1967;54:167-179.

Walker AM & Rothman KJ. Models of varying parametric form in case-referent studies. *American Journal of Epidemiology* 1982;115:129-137.

Woolf B. On estimating the relation between blood group and disease. *Annals of Human Genetics* 1955;19:251-253.

Zelen M. The analysis of several 2 × 2 contingency tables. *Biometrika* 1971; 58:129-137.

INDEX